MW01255014

Chinese Medicinal Wines & Elixirs

by
Bob
Flaws

✽ BLUE POPPY PRESS

Published by:

BLUE POPPY PRESS, INC.
1775 LINDEN AVE.
BOULDER, CO 80304

First Edition, September 1994
Second Printing , October 1997

ISBN 0-936185-58-9
LC 94-77988

The information in this book is given in good faith. However, the translators and the publishers cannot be held responsible for any error or omission. Nor can they be held in any way responsible for treatment given on the basis of information contained in this book. The publishers make this information available to English language readers for scholarly and research purposes only.

The publishers do not advocate nor endorse self-medication by laypersons. Chinese medicine is a professional medicine. Laypersons interested in availing themselves of the treatments described in this book should seek out a qualified professional practitioner of Chinese medicine.

COMP Designation: Original compilation based on Chinese sources

Printed at Bookcrafters, Chelsea, MI
on chlorine-free paper

10 9 8 7 6 5 4 3 2

Preface

This book is based on a number of Chinese sources, both premodern and contemporary. The main premodern sources include the *Ben Cao Gang Mu (Complete Outline of the Materia Medica)*, the *Wan Bing Hui Chun (Returning Spring to Ten Thousand Diseases)*, the *Gu Jin Yi Tong Da Quan (A Large [i.e., Comprehensive] Collection of Medicine Past & Present)*, the *Yan Fang Xin Bian (New Compilation of Time-tested Formulas)*, the *Tai Ping Sheng Hui Fang (The Supreme Peace Holy & Benevolent Formulas)*, the *Sheng Ji Zong Lu (General Collection for Holy Relief)*, and the *Qian Jin Fang (Thousand [Ducats] of Gold Formulas)*. Contemporary Chinese sources include the *Zhong Guo Yi Xue Da Ci Dian (Encyclopedia of Medicine in China)* published by the Shanghai Science & Technology Press, *Zhong Hua Shi Wu Liao Fa Da Quan (A Large [i.e., Comprehensive] Collection of Chinese Food Treatments)* published by the Jiangsu Science & Technology Press, *Zhong Yi Shang Ke Xue (TCM Traumatology)* also published by Shanghai Science & Technology Press, *Zhong Yi Wai Ke Xue (The Study of TCM External Medicine)* published by the People's Press, *Zhong Guo Zhong Yi Mi Fang Da Quan (A Complete Collection of TCM Secret Formulas in China)* compiled by Hu Xi-ming, *Jia Ting Yao Jiu (Family Lineage Medicinal Wines)*, by Hao Shou-zhou *et.al.*, published by Whole Shield Press, Beijing, and, especially for folk prescriptions and the general organization of the formulas in this book, the *Yao Jiu Yan Fang Jiang (A Selection of Effective Medicinal Wine Formulas)* by Sun Wen-qi published by China Books Press in Hong Kong in 1986. English language sources include Sung Baek's Chinese herbal medicine course sponsored by Oriental Medical Research Inc. of Chicago and Henry C. Lu's *Chinese System of Food Cures: Prevention & Remedies*.

Material compiled from Chinese sources was functionally translated using Nigel Wiseman's standard terminology as appearing in a *Glossary of Chinese Medical Terms & Acupuncture Points* published by Paradigm Books, Brookline, MA. The exception to this is that I have used network vessels to translate *luo* (络) instead of connecting vessels as it appears in that glossary. This change is based on a revised list of terms supplied to me by Nigel Wiseman. Medicinal identifications are based on Bensky & Gamble's *Chinese Herbal Medicine: Materia Medica*; Hong-yen Hsu's *Oriental Materia Medica: A Concise Guide*; G.A. Stuart *et al.*'s *Chinese Materia Medica*; and the *Zhong Yao Da Ci Dian (Encyclopedia of Chinese Medicinals)*.

Bob Flaws
September 1, 1994

Table of Contents

1

Introduction

On the cover of this book is a picture of a gourd. Called a *hu lu* in Chinese and a bottle gourd in English, such a gourd is a common iconographic accoutrement of Daoist immortals and itinerant Chinese doctors in Old China for it is the symbol of the elixir of immortality. So closely is this bottle gourd holding a medicinal elixir associated with Chinese medicine that the *hu lu* is the symbol of the traditional Chinese doctor the way the caduceus is the symbol of a Western medical doctor. On this *hu lu* are the words "Compassionate Art", referring to the practice of medicine.

In addition, the complicated or old character for writing the word medicine in Chinese, *yi* (醫) contains the bottle radical (酉) as a component in its lower half. This bottle radical itself is a stylized representation of a bottle with wine in it. This goes to show that the use of medicinal wines is very old within Chinese medicine and is integral to its practice.

In Chinese, the character *jiu* (酒) refers to any type of alcoholic drink. This includes wines, "sherries" and "brandies", and distilled liquors. As mentioned above, within Traditional Chinese Medicine, there is a long history of using medicines made in the form of wines, liqueurs, and spirituous beverages. Generically, these are referred to as *yao jiu*, medicinal wines. A short history of the use and development of Chinese medicinal wines is given in the following chapter.

In Chinese medicine, there are two basic ways of making such medicinal wines. The first is to actually ferment the medicinal ingredients. This is the more traditional or ancient method. However, because this is a time-consuming and relatively complex procedure, a simpler method has been used since the advent of distilled liquors. This is to simply soak the medicinal ingredients in alcohol, thus making what is technically referred to as a tincture.

Types of Chinese "Wines"

There are several different types of wines and distilled spirits used in making the Chinese medicinal wines described in this book. These include:

1) *Huang jiu* or yellow wine. This refers to wine made out of rice or millet. This is similar to Japanese sake and sake may be used as a substitute for Chinese yellow wine in making Chinese medicinal wines in the West.

2) *Pu tao jiu* or grape wine. In China, this usually means red wine. Although this type of wine is not used so frequently in making Chinese medicinal wines, it is sometimes used.

3) *Bai jiu* or white alcohol. This refers to any distilled grain alcohol. The alcoholic content of a *bai jiu* is much higher than a yellow or rice wine. In the Chinese medical literature, *bai jiu* is also called *qing jiu* or clear alcohol. Likewise, it may also be called *hao jiu*, good or unadulterated alcohol, or *chun jiu*, mellow, good, unadulterated alcohol.

4) *Gao liang jiu* is a type of very strong, distilled, clear alcohol made from sorghum. This can be bought in Chinese-owned liquor stores in Western Chinatowns. This is really only a type of *bai jiu*.

Because *pu tao jiu* and *gao liang jiu* are only varieties of wine and grain alcohol respectively, Henry C. Lu, author of *Chinese System of Food Cures*, says that there are two types of alcohol used to make Chinese medicinal wines, rice wine and white alcohol.

Who Typically Uses Medicinal Wines in China

Medicinal wines are mostly used during the winter months and also by older patients. As we will see below, a *little* alcohol warms the center and supplements the qi while at the same time it raises clear yang and quickens the blood. In older patients, spleen and stomach function is typically weak and taking one's medicine as a medicated wine helps improve this situation. Likewise, older patients commonly have poor circulation. On the one hand, this means they often have cold feet or cold hands and feet. On the other, their diseases are often complicated by an element of stasis and stagnation which a *little* alcohol helps address. For instance, a large number of the medicinal wines are for the treatment of rheumatism and arthritis in the elderly. Taking medicinal wines is very good for treating such conditions.

In addition, many chronic conditions require the taking of medicine over a prolonged period of time. Cooking and taking decoctions day in and day out can, therefore, become an onerous chore, whereas, taking a nip of medicinal wine is quick, easy, and enjoyable. Because a little alcohol is good for the elderly's digestion, especially in the winter, medicinal wines may also be easier on the stomach and easier to digest than medicated pills and powders.

Further, medicinal wines are typically more concentrated and potent than decoctions and pills. Therefore, they are especially useful for treating post-stroke patients whose ability to drink large quantities of liquids may be impaired.

Who Should Not Use Chinese Medicinal Wines

Generally, young and middle-aged adults should not make much use of Chinese medicinal wines. Although the young (and especially young martial artists) may be fascinated by the idea of supplementing their qi and strengthening their sinews and bones, wine, as we will see below, is a toxic food. It should not be used inappropriately or in excess. Likewise, as Zhang Zi-he, one of the four great masters of internal medicine of the Jin-Yuan Dynasties said, taking supplements without having a true vacuity or deficiency only causes illness. It is important not to try to gild the lily. Young and middle-aged adults usually have plenty of qi. In fact, most often their diseases and complaints are due to an inability to circulate the qi they have or are due to too much heat in their bodies.

In addition, patients suffering from polysystemic chronic candidiasis or from diabetes mellitus should use Chinese medicated wines with extreme care. Since most patients with rheumatoid arthritis (as opposed to rheumatic or osteoarthritis) do exhibit signs and symptoms of systemic candidiasis, they typically should not attempt to use the medicinal wines in this book. This also goes for sufferers of lupus erythematosus and multiple sclerosis or anyone suffering from an immune deficiency or autoimmune disorder.

Categories of *Yao Jiu*

There are several different categories of Chinese medicinal wines described in this book. These include wines for:

1) Supplementing vacuity detriment. This means wines for the treatment of various deficiency and debility conditions commonly encountered in the elderly or chronically ill.

2) Strengthening the sinews and bones. This refers to wines which nourish the liver and supplement the kidneys and thus strengthen the sinews and bones. Weakness of the sinews and bones is another of the conditions most frequently encountered among older patients.

3) Dispelling wind. These wines all treat wind damp *bi* or rheumatic and arthritic conditions.

4) Clearing heat and disinhibiting dampness. The wines in this category treat inflammatory conditions due to damp heat. This includes red, swollen eyes, oral sores and bleeding gums, inhibited urination, foot qi, lung abscess, dysentery, summerheat, jaundice, etc.

5) Fortifying the spleen and harmonizing the stomach. These wines all help to supplement the spleen. Simply put, this means they aid digestion. As stated above, one of the effects of aging is the weakening of the digestion. This means that older patients often suffer from digestive complaints, such as vomiting, diarrhea, abdominal distention after meals, hiccup, belching and acid regurgitation, etc. It also means older patients may be prone to lack of appetite with consequent weight loss and fatigue.

6) Gynecological wines. The wines in this section all treat various menstrual irregularities and pre- and postpartum complaints.

7) External invasion, damage by wind. The wines in this section treat flus and the common cold. Such wines can be made in advance and be stored indefinitely. Therefore, Chinese medicated wines can be a very effective and pragmatic treatment for the first inklings of a common cold.

8) Wines for warding off scourges. Scourges refer to pestilential disease. The wines in this category help prevent the catching of warm, seasonal, epidemic diseases.

9) Traumatic injury. Traumatic injury typically involves qi stagnation and blood stasis with accumulation of depressive heat and obstruction of body fluids. Because alcohol quickens the blood and thus helps to transform or dispel stasis, medicinal wines are effective for treating many kinds of traumatic injury. In addition, they can be prepared beforehand and stored indefinitely until called for by accident or emergency.

10) *Pao zhen* or herpes. The wines in this chapter all deal with various types of skin rashes. In particular, herpes zoster is more prevalent in the elderly because, according to modern Western medicine, the typically weakened immune system in the elderly or chronically ill can no longer suppress the virus. If seen as a deep-lying warm evil (*fu wen xie*) according to TCM theory, the expression of these damp heat evil toxins in the elderly is due to a decline and exhaustion of *jing* essence.

11) Miscellaneous wines. The medicinal wines in this chapter cover all variety of diseases, including respiratory diseases, parasites, deafness and ringing in the ears, etc.

The TCM Description of Alcohol as a Medicinal Substance

According to Chinese books on food therapy, *jiu* or alcohol is bitter, sweet, and acrid in flavor. It is warm in nature and it is also toxic. It enters the channels of the heart, liver, lungs, and stomach. In terms of its medicinal functions, alcohol opens the blood vessels, wards off cold qi, arouses the spleen and warms the center, and moves (*i.e.*, makes more capable) the power of medicinals. Alcohol's qi is also upbearing and outwardly dispersing. In clinical practice, alcohol mainly is used to treat wind cold *bi* pain, contracture and spasm of the sinews and vessels, chest *bi*, and chilly pain in the heart and abdomen.

Alcohol by itself is generally contraindicated for those suffering from yin vacuity or serious damp heat patterns and also for those who have recently lost a lot of blood. Although medicinal wines may be used in cases of yin vacuity and damp heat, they should still be used with care. In general, Chinese medicinal wines are mainly and most safely used for the treatment of cold patterns rather than either vacuity or repletion heat patterns.

In the late nineteenth century, Jin Zi-jiu wrote a somewhat different description of alcohol emphasizing its negative qualities. Jin Zi-jiu says:

> Alcohol has a volatile nature that damages the spirit and injures the blood. Its qi is hot and it leads to waste and decline. Alcohol first enters the gallbladder and liver where gallbladder fire explodes. The qi loses its restraint and descension. Liver yin is looted. The blood becomes unsettled and, as a result, counterflow upbearing with vomiting of blood can occur. Moreover, alcohol is damp as well as hot. Dampness injures the spleen. This creates stagnant food and phlegm which easily gum up the qi mechanism. Heat damages the lungs and easily causes coughing and wheezing. If chronically vacuous with no recovery, lung damage eventually affects the kidneys. The kidneys are the water viscus and once kidney water is vacuous, the five ministerial fires increase many fold, wiping out qi and *ying*. In short, ... drinking damages the blood.[1]

Therefore, when using alcohol, it is important to remember that its nature is upbearing and dispersing, heating and also dampening. Small amounts arouse the spleen but large amounts result in damaging the

---

[1] Jiu Zi-jiu, *Jin Zi Jiu Zhuan Ji (A Collection of Jin Zi-jiu's Expertise)*, Peoples's Health & Hygiene Press, Beijing, 1982, p. 85-6

spleen. Small amounts quicken the blood, but large amounts damage the blood. Small amounts scatter cold and warm the center, but large amounts stir ministerial fire. And further, it should be remembered that alcohol is toxic in the TCM sense. Like many other TCM medicinals, alcohol is not safe in an of itself. It is very powerful. That power can be used for good in small amounts or for bad in large amounts. Therefore, the reader will see that many of the discussions of medicinal wines in this book end with the injunction that their use should be suspended when the condition is cured or that they should not be drunk to excess.

The Unique Repertoire of Chinese Medicinals Used in Medicinal Wines

Those readers familiar with Chinese medicinals in general and with Chinese medicinals typically prescribed in decoctions in particular will note that many of the Chinese medicinals used over and over again in the formulas in this book are not commonly prescribed in decoction. Thus one can say that there is a seemingly special *materia medica* used in Chinese medicinal wines. This includes ingredients such as Fructus Zanthoxyli Bungeani (*Chuan Jiao* or *Shu Jiao*) and Herba Cum Radice Asari (*Xi Xin*). Both these ingredients are very pungent, penetrating, and dispersing. Thus they work well with alcohol's pungent, penetrating, dispersing nature. Likewise the reader will see that Radix Praeparatus Aconiti Carmichaeli (*Fu Zi*) and Cortex Cinnamomi (*Rou Gui, Gui Xin*, or *Guan Gui*) are used exceedingly often in the formulas in this book. These are the two most important warming medicinals in the Chinese *materia medica* and thus they too complement alcohol's warm nature. In addition, their common use is based on the fact that Chinese medicinal wines are used to primarily treat cold patterns.

Another ingredient that is commonly found in formulas in this book but not so commonly found is decocted formulas in Herba Dendrobii (*Shi Hu*). This medicinal is a yin supplement which in particular nourishes stomach yin fluids. I believe this ingredient is used so often in Chinese medicinal wines for two reasons. First, stomach yin vacuity is a common complicating pattern in the elderly and Chinese medicinal wines are most often used by older patients. Secondly, alcohol being hot in nature easily damages and exhausts yin fluids in the stomach. The addition of Herba Dendrobii helps to prevent that from happening.

There are also some ingredients which turn up time and again in these formulas which are hardly every come across in standard decoction formulas. These include Caulis et Folium Skimmiae Reevesianae (*Yin Yu*), Caulis et Folium Sambucudis Javanicae (*Lu Ying*), and various parts of the pine tree: Nodus Pini (*Song Jie*), Folium Pini (*Song Ye*), and Radix Pini (*Song Gen*). The resins in pine have been used to quicken the blood and penetrate stasis in many cultures. They also go into solution in alcohol much easier than in water. Thus it is not surprising that they show up so often in formulas meant to treat traumatic injury and *bi* pathoconditions. As for the Sambucus, it is a specific for the treatment of wind damp *bi* and traumatic injury. Because many of these formulas are folk formulas and because Elder can be found growing locally, it was/is an easy medicinal to get as are pine needles and wood. Likewise, the Skimmia is also a specific antirheumatic. However, because it enters the liver and kidney channels and treats debility and weakness of the legs and feet and not just wind dampness, it also would be especially effective in the treatment of older patients who tend to be liver/kidney vacuous and deficient.

2

The History of Medicinal Wines in China

The earliest written record of wine-making in China comes from the Warring States period (476-221 BCE). In a political history of that time, it is said:

> Once upon a time, the Heavenly Princess ordered Yi Di to make wine and present it to Yu (the first king of China and founder of the Xia Dynasty [2205-1766 BCE]). Yu drank it and enjoyed its sweetness.

Thus Yi Di is credited as the first wine-maker in Chinese history. However, a better known wine-maker was Du Kang, a fifth generation descendant of Yu. His name is often used as a historical allusion to wine in Chinese and is also incorporated in the logos of several modern Chinese distilleries. For instance, in a famous poem by Cao Cao, a.k.a. Cao Meng-de, the infamous dictator of the Three Kingdoms period (220-280 CE), there is a couplet which goes,

> What will resolve my worries?
> Nothing other than Du Kang.

From the Shang Dynasty (1766-1122 BCE), the knowledge and practice of wine-making spread across China. In the *Shang Shu (History of the Shang)*, Wu Ding, a king of the Shang Dynasty, said, "If sweet wine is to be made, distiller's yeast should be used." This statement suggests that wine-making had already reached a high level of sophistication by that time. It is also interesting to note that the majority of bronze vessels unearthed from the Yin ruins dating from the Shang Dynasty are either production vessels for the manufacture of wine or vessels for its storage. During this dynasty, wine was not only a popular drink but also an important item of sacrifice in religious rituals. Inscriptions on bones and shells dating from this period describe the brewing of a special wine used for sacrifice from various kinds of herbs mixed with aromatic tumeric. It is quite possible that this herbal wine was not only used for religious sacrifices but also had some medicinal application.

During the Zhou Dynasty (1122-256 BCE), a special government body was set up which was in charge of wine production. Further, wine-making techniques and production methods are described in detail in the *Zhou Li (Rituals of Zhou)*. According to this book, there were six principles for making high quality wine. These included the use of pure water, high quality raw materials, appropriate tools, and the right processing methods.

In the Western Zhou Dynasty (1122-771 BCE), the practice of medicine within the royal palace was divided into four departments. Thus there were food or dietary physicians, disease physicians, trauma physicians, and veterinary physicians. In particular, there were two dietary doctors who were in charge of the arrangement of the "six foods, six beverages, and six dishes" for the king. Wine was among these six beverages. Therefore, it is apparent that prescribing wine as a medicine was practiced at the court as early as the Western Zhou. This was called *yao jiu* or medicinal wine and was used both to protect health and to cure illness.

The oldest formulas for the brewing of *yao jiu* or Chinese medicinal wines are found in two books discovered in 1973 in the tomb of King Ma. These two books are the *Yang Sheng Fang (Formulas for Nourishing Life)* and *Za Liao Fang (Formulas for Treating Miscellaneous [Diseases])*. Only one *yao jiu* formula is found in the *Zao Liao Fang*, but six are found in the *Yang Sheng Fang*. These include wine made from Tuber Ophiopogonis Japonicae (*Mai Men Dong*) and sorghum; wine made from glutinous millet and glutinous rice; a mellow wine made from wheat; wine made from Gypsum Fibrosum (*Shi Gao*), Radix Et Rhizoma Ligustici Chinensis (*Gao Ben*), and Radix Achyranthis Bidentatae (*Niu Xi*); wine made from Lacca Exsiccata Sinica (*Qi*) and Radix Aconiti (*Wu Tou*); and wine made from Lacca Exsiccata Sinica (*Qi*), glutinous millet, rice, Radix Aconiti (*Wu Tou*), and Rhizoma Polygonati Odorati (*Yu Zhu*). In some formulas from the *Yang Sheng Fang*, not only are the ingredients listed but the brewing process, method of administration, and indications are all also discussed in detail.

The *Huang Di Nei Jing (Yellow Emperor's Inner Classic)* is the single most important book in the development of Traditional Chinese Medicine or TCM. Although it came to relative completion in the Han Dynasty (206 BCE-220 CE), it was, in fact, largely the product of pre-Qin (221-206 BCE) knowledge. In this preeminent classic there is a chapter titled *"Tang Ye Liao Li Lun* (Treatise on Fluids, Turbid Wine & Fragrant Wine)." One should note that fluids as used in this instance is a collective term for wines. In this chapter it specifies that medicinal wine should be made "with rice (as the raw material) and rice stalks as the fuel (in processing) because rice is lacking in nothing (in terms of qi), while its stalks are strong (for fueling a fire)." Then it proceeds:

> Sages in ancient times prepared fluids, turbid and fragrant wines just in case of (unusual) need... Since the medieval ages, morals began to deteriorate and evil qi frequently came. Then, taking (medicinal wines) became a cure-all remedy.

Bian Que, who is believed to have lived during the 5th century BCE, is the first Chinese doctor for whom we have a written biography. In Si-ma Qian's *Shi Ji (The History)* in which Bian Que's biography is found, the author devotes some space to Bian Que's views on medicinal wines and their treatment efficacy. This further verifies the development of medicinal wines in the pre-Qin period.

13

In the Han Dynasty, there was great development in Chinese medicine with many preeminent physicians. These included Hua Tuo, Zhang Zhong-jing, and Cang Gong, a.k.a. Chun Yu-yi. In Chun Yu-yi's collection of 25 case histories, the first in Chinese medicine and appearing in the *Shi Ji*, there are two cases treated with *yao jiu* or medicinal wines. One was the Prince of Ji Bei who suffered from aversion to wind with chest fullness. He was cured by Chun using *San Shi Yao Jiu* (Three Stones Medicinal Wine). The other case was of a lady named Wang. She suffered from difficult delivery and was relieved by a wine made from black henbane. In addition, this wine helped save the baby.

In his *Shang Han Lun/Jin Gui Yao Lue (Treatise on Cold Damage/Formulas from the Golden Cabinet),* Zhang Zhong-jing (150-219 CE) gives no lack of discussions on how to cook medicinal wines, how to administer prepared medicinals together with wine, and how to treat disease with medicinal wines. For instance, Zhang suggests, "For the 62 winds in females with qi and blood pricking pain in the abdomen, *Hong Lan Hua Jiu* (Safflower Wine) is the ruling remedy." This formula is still in use today and is given in this present work.

During the Sui and Tang Dynasties (589-907 CE), the use of medicinal wines increased dramatically. In Sun Si-miao's *Qian Jin Yao Fang (Formulas [Worth] a Thousand [Pieces of] Gold)*, there are 80 formulas for various *yao jiu*. These are indicated for *nei ke* (internal medicine), *wai ke* (external medicine), and *fu ke* (gynecological) diseases as well as for supplementing vacuity and nourishing life. In a companion volume (*Qian Jin Yi Fang*), Sun included a separate chapter on medicinal wines in which he discusses 200 wine formulas. This is the first individual essay on medicinal wines in Chinese history. However, Sun also recognized the deleterious effects of drinking too much wine and also wrote the first TCM description of wine's ill effects. Based on Sun's views, many Chinese doctors began designing and researching treatments for alcohol intoxication, wine toxins, and other alcohol-related symptoms.

In the Song through Yuan Dynasties (969-1368 CE), wine production became a prosperous industry due to certain advances in technology. Because wines and alcohol became all the more available and widespread, Chinese doctors devoted more time to discussing and researching wine and alcohol's effects on the human body. Therefore, during this period, many books on wine and alcohol were published. As far back as the Tang Dynasty, a book titled the *Jiu Jing (Wine Classic)* had been published, and in the Song Dynasty, several more books bearing the same title were published. Even Su Shi, the most famous poet of this period, wrote a book titled the *Wine Classic*. However, it was the eminent physician Zhu Hong, author of the *Hui Ren Shu (Book of Rescuing People)*, who contributed the most to medicinal wine research during this period. In his *Bei Shan Jiu Jing (Wine Classic of the Northern Mountain)*, Zhu discussed every aspect of wine and alcohol, including processing methods, yeast cultivation, and sterilization by heating.

Thus during this period, people in China began to have a fuller understanding of alcohol in terms of its actions and medicinal applications. In the *Tai Ping Sheng Hui Fang (Holy & Benevolent Formulas from the Tai Ping [Reign])*, it is stated:

> Wine, the essence of grain, harmonizes and nourishes the spirit and qi. However, since it is swift and fierce by nature, it may work in a precarious way. It is capable of perfusing and disinhibiting the stomach and intestines and is good at conducting the force of (other) medicinals.

In another book of this period, the *Sheng Ji Zong Lu ([His] Majesty's General Records of [Our] Ancestors)*, it is stated:

Evils may bring people either shallow or deep damage, and medicinals may attack evils with either light or serious momentum. At the initial stage of disease, one should treat the fine problems with liquids (*i.e.*, decoctions). When the illness has lasted for a long time, (however,) one should administer turbid and fragrant wine to attack the grave problem. There are also cases of the forms having experienced frequent fright and shock and of blocked channels and network vessels, a disease resulting in insensitivity. (To treat such cases,) the medicinals should be processed with alcohol. Because such cases suffer from evils which have penetrated deeply and the channels and vessels are stopped and stagnated, nothing other than medicinal wine, which disperses and diffuses evil qi, perfuses and frees the vessels, can cure them... Because wine is tremendously hot in nature and, therefore, can immediately convey the heat of medicinals, it is proper for patients to take it constantly who suffer from blood vacuity and stagnant qi, long-standing cold and inveterate frigidity, hemilateral withering with paraplegia, hypertonicity, *bi*, inversion, and the like. This makes use of wine's gradual force of steeping. In addition, according to ancient methodology, medicinals were usually administered along with wine. This was not merely for the purpose of diffusing and freeing blood and qi but also nourishes yang.

In the prescriptions predating that period, medicinal wines were indicated for a comparatively small number of conditions. These included wind patterns, such as wind aching and pain in the low back and legs for instance. However, from this time, the scope of application of medicinal wines increased progressively so that it was not only used to treat disease but also to preserve health, extend longevity, and improve one's beauty. At the same time, more and more medicinals were used as ingredients in medicinal wine. In the *Wine Classic of the Northern Mountain* alone, 13 medicinals are recorded. For instance, in *Xiang Gui Jiu* (Fragrant Cinnamon Wine), the mash is composed of Cortex Cinnamomi (*Guan Gui*), Radix Ledebouriellae Sesloidis (*Fang Feng*), Radix Saussureae Seu Vladimiriae (*Mu Xiang*), and Semen Pruni Armeniacae (*Xing Ren*). Also, physicians of this period

16

paid attention to the quality of the tincturing alcohol, with Dong Yang wine being given special credit. This wine was said to have a fresh scent which could reach far, was a golden color, and caused no bad side effects, such as headache, thirst, or diarrhea. Likewise, it was believed that the water used in making medicinal wines should have a good flavor and be "heavier" than water found in most places.

As the production of medicinal wines continued to develop, their popularity increased. This is because they not only preserved health and cured disease but were also mellow and good-tasting. Thus medicinal wines entered the palace as tribute from the provinces. During the Yuan Dynasty (1280-1368 CE), *Gou Qi Jiu* (Lycium Wine) and *Di Huang Jiu* (Rehmannia Wine) came from the northwest of China. *Lu Rong Jiu* (Deer Antler Wine) and *Song Jie Jiu* (Pine Node Wine) came from northeast China. *Fu Ling Jiu* (Poria Wine) came from south China. And *Hei Ji Jiu* (Black Chicken Wine) and *Hai Gou Shen* (Seal Genitals Wine) came from southwest China.

In the Ming Dynasty (1368-1644 CE), most of the emperors dissipated themselves in wine and sex, and among the most popular wines were *yao jiu* or medicinal wines. One of the emperors' favorite wines was made with Rhizoma Atractylodis Macrocephalae (*Bai Zhu*), Lignum Santali Albi (*Bai Tan Xiang*), Fructus Amomi (*Sha Ren*), Herba Agastachis Seu Pogostemmi (*Huo Xiang*), Radix Glycyrrhizae (*Gan Cao*), Radix Saussureae Seu Vladimiriae (*Mu Xiang*), and Flos Caryophylli (*Ding Xiang*). Such fondness for wine and alcohol was not confined to the imperial palace, and distilleries sprang up around the country supplying medicinal wines to the common people. In addition, the custom sprang up that people made medicinal wines at home which they drank on certain holidays each year. Thus, on the fifth day of the fifth month, people drank *Chang Pu Jiu* (Acorus Wine), while at the Mid-autumn Festival, *Gui Hua Jiu* (Osmanthus Flower Wine) was a treat.

17

Also in the Ming Dynasty, Li Shi-zhen, in his monumental *Ben Cao Gang Mu (Great Outline of Materia Medica)*, further established wine or alcohol's TCM medicinal description:

> Wine's nature is pure yang and its flavor is acrid and sweet. It upbears yang, effuses, and scatters, and its qi is dry and hot. It overcomes dampness and expels cold...

> Wine, a beauty bestowed by heaven—drinking a small amount harmonizes the blood and moves the qi, strengthens the spirit and wards off cold, disperses worry and dispels moodiness. Drinking a painful (*i.e.*, extreme or pathological) amount damages the spirit and consumes the blood, causes detriment to the stomach and death to the essence, engenders phlegm and stirs fire... Addiction to wine and getting drunk on a regular basis leads to disease and decay at best and to humiliation of one's nation, ruination of one's family, and loss of one's life at worst.

During these early dynasties, medicinal wines were made by fermenting the medicinal ingredients right in the mash. However, by the early Qing Dynasty (1644-1911 CE), alcohol was being commercially distilled and allowed for the tincturing of medicinals in ready-made, store bought alcohol. These kinds of medicinal wines were usually spoken of as *gan lu* or dew. This meant that they were a sweet-smelling beverage made with fragrant fruits and flowers. The most common of these were Rose Dew, Lotus Flower Dew, and Hawthorne Berry Dew. Because such medicinal wines were designed to protect the origin and solidify the root, contribute to longevity and prolong one's years, they were extremely popular with the rich and well-to-do. At this time, the capital, Peking, was the center of the medicinal wine industry. The following poem from that time describes this vibrant industry:

> Brewhouses can be seen abutted by low walls
> Extending to the horizon in the distance,
> Standing in line from the Forbidden City to the brink of the water.

Flowers in season are brought in time for brewing wine.
Through the bamboo forest, breezes send the fragrance of wine.

During the reign of the Guo Min Tang (KMT), the making of medicinal wines as with the practice of Traditional Chinese Medicine in general went into decline. However, shortly after the Chinese Communist take-over, Mao Ze-dong encouraged the revitalization of TCM as a national treasure trove worthy of research and promulgation. Since that time, numerous special TCM research institutes, colleges, and hospitals have been established. In this milieu of renewed interest in all things TCM, Chinese medicinal wines have likewise received renewed research and interest. There are numerous Chinese medicinal wines now manufactured in the People's Republic of China and distributed both domestically and internationally. Chinese medicinal wines have been included in the State Pharmacopeia and there is a move toward their standardization in terms of production, quality, indications, and administration.

Nonetheless, Chinese medicinal wines can be made simply and easily by anyone with access to the ingredients. As seen above, medicinal wines have a very long history in China. Hopefully, this book will help establish the manufacture and use of Chinese medicinal wines in the West.

3

Basic Instructions

General Instructions on Making Chinese Medicinal Wines

As the reader will see, there are several different types of instructions in the formulas given below. This is because these formulas have been taken from a number of different sources. I have not given any formulas that require actually fermenting Chinese medicinals to produce a wine. All the formulas in this book are made using ready-made, commercially available wines and spirits. In general, one puts a specified amount of Chinese medicinals in a jar and then allows this to soak or tincture in a specified amount and type of alcohol for a specified length of time.

The amount of time the tincture must sit depends on the nature of the medicinal ingredients, such as how quickly and easily their active ingredients enter solution, and the coarseness of their cut. If one uses large pieces or chunks of herbal roots and barks or large chunks of stones or shells, the time required for the tincture to sit is typically 1 month. If, however, one grinds the ingredients into powder, the time required to make a medicinal tincture is reduced to a matter of 3-7 days.

When discussing the method of preparation of many of the formulas given in this book that specify that the medicinal ingredients are to be ground into either a coarse or fine powder, there is also the instruction that the resulting powder should be wrapped in a cloth bag. This makes it much easier to remove the dregs from the resulting tincture.

Even in cases where this instruction is not given, the reader should consider doing this. It can make the manufacture of such tincture much cleaner and simpler. However, if one does this, they should shake the jar at least once per day.

The reader will also see that some tinctures are made quite quickly by putting the jar containing the alcohol and medicinals in a pan of water and bringing it to a boil one or several times in succession. Using this method, one can make a tincture in several hours rather than several days or a month.

In formulas that specify white or clear alcohol, one can use either vodka or grain alcohol. *Be absolutely certain not to use rubbing or wood alcohol!* These are poisonous and should not be used for any medicinal wine meant for internal consumption. If the taste of such high proof clear spirits is too strong for the patient, one can add either honey or sugar to the alcohol to make it more palatable or one can use a strong brandy or cognac. However, one should definitely not add honey or sugar or use brandy or cognac in patients who are either hyper- or hypoglycemic.

General Instructions for Taking Chinese Medicinal Wines

Under each formula in this book there is a heading for method of administration. Under this heading, the reader will find the recommended dosage for each formula. The dosages are generally given in either milliliters (ml) or in terms of Chinese teacups. A Chinese teacup is smaller than a Western measuring cup and usually smaller than even the typical Western, handled tea or coffee cup. When the instructions say a small teacup, they are referring to something the size of what we in the West refer to as a shot glass.

Most of the formulas in this book specify how many times per day to take each formula. Sometimes it is specified to take the formula in the morning and evening. Sometimes it is specified to take the formula morning, noon, and night. Sometimes it is specified to take the formula either before or after meals or on an empty stomach. And sometimes it is specified that the formula should be drunk warm.

In some cases, there is no set time or set amount. The reader is advised to use the formula as necessary. Sometimes such formulas say to take a suitable amount and sometimes they say to take as much as one wants. Frequently, the instructions say that one should feel the qi of the alcohol or just slightly tipsy or high. However, one should not drink any of these formulas to the point of outright drunkenness.

Converting Measurements

Most of the formulas in this book say to use so many *jin* of this or that type of alcohol. A *jin* is a traditional Chinese measure of weight. One *jin* equals 17.6 oz. *avdp.* (not fluid ounces). One *jin* also equals 0.5 kg. One must weigh the alcohol in formulas which are given in *jin*. Other formulas say to use so many milliliters (ml) of alcohol. Milliliter and liters are both measurements of volume, not weight. One cup equals 236.6ml. According to *A Barefoot Doctor's Manual, Revised & Enlarged Edition*, 1ml also equals 1cc, and some of the formulas in this book say to use so many cc's of alcohol.[1] Another way of thinking about this is that 1 gal. (US) consists of 3785ml and 1 gal. (Imp.) equals 4740ml. One gal. equals 4 quarts. Of course 1000ml equals 1 liter.

---

[1] *A Barefoot Doctor's Manual*, Revised & Enlarged Edition, Cloudburst Press, Mayne Isle & Seattle, 1977, inside back cover

Most of the medicinals in formulas in this book are given in terms of grams (g). There are 28.4g in 1 oz. and 453.6g in 1 lb.

These conversions should allow Westerners to figure out the dosages in the formulas in this book according to whatever system they are most familiar. Commonly, electronic kitchen scales for weighing out foods and spices can read in either ounces or grams. I believe such scales are the easiest and best for weighing out Chinese medicinals in the West.

Obtaining the Ingredients

Readers in the United States can order most of the Chinese medicinals mentioned in this book from:

Spring Wind Herb Company
2315 Fourth St.
Berkeley, CA 94710
Tel. 510-849-1820
1-800-588-4883

This company sells Chinese herbs by mail order and customers can order using either the Pinyin romanization of the Chinese name or the Latin pharmacological name. (I give both in this book.) This company goes to great lengths to import and sell Chinese herbs free from pesticides, fumigants, bleaches, and other chemical contaminants.

Other companies in the United States that sell Chinese herbs by mail are:

China Herb Co.
165 W. Queen Lane
Philadelphia, PA 19144

Tel. 215-843-5864, 800-221-4372; Fax 215-849-3338

Mayway Corp.
1338 Cypress St.
Oakland, CA 94607
Tel. 510-208-3113

North South China Herbs Co.
1556 Stockton Street
San Francisco, CA 94133
Tel. 415-421-4907

Nuherbs Co.
3820 Penniman Avenue
Oakland, CA 94619
Tel. 415-534-4372; 800-233-4307

For those in the United Kingdom, most of the medicinals in this book
can be ordered from:

Acumedic Ltd.
101-105 Camden High Street
London NW1 7JN
Tel. 071-388-6704/5783; Fax 071-387-5766

East West Herb Shop
3 Neals Yard
Covent Garden, London WC2H 9DP
Tel. 071-379-1312; Fax 071-379-4414

Harmony Acupuncture Supplies Center
629 High Road Leytonstone
London E11 4PA
Tel. 081-518-7337; Fax 081-518-7338

Mayway Herbal Emporium
40 Sapcote Trading Estate, Dudden Hill Lane
London NW10 2DJ
Tel. 081-459-1812; Fax 081-459-1727

For those in Europe, most of the medicinals in this book can be ordered from:

Homeofar n.v.
Hugo Verriestlaan 63
8500 Kortrijk, Belgium

Tai Yang Chinese Herb Store
Elverdingsestr. 90A
8900 Ieper, Belgium
Tel. 057-21-86-69; Fax 057-21-97-78

Apotheek Gouka
Goenelaan 111
3114 CE Schiedam, Netherlands
Tel. 010-426-46-33; Fax 010-473-08-45

And for those in Australia, most of the medicinals in this book can be ordered from:

Chinaherb
29A Albion St.
Surry Hills, NSW 2010
Tel. 02-281-2122

What to Do If You Cannot Find an Ingredient

As discussed above in the introduction, some of the medicinals used in Chinese *yao jiu* are unusual when compared to those used in standard decoctions. Therefore, depending on the supplier, some of the ingredients which would be locally available to Chinese folk in the countryside may not be available from Chinese herb suppliers and importers. In that case, what should the practitioner do who is trying to make one of these medicinal wines for a patient?

First of all, there is nothing sacred or inviolable about these formulas. They were created by human beings just like ourselves. As the reader will see, there are numerous formulas which are quite similar except for one or two ingredients and they still accomplish the same therapeutic goals. In Chinese clinics, if the dispensary is out of an ingredient prescribed by a doctor, the prescription is sent back upstairs and the practitioner is asked to choose something else in its place. In this case, the practitioner must first identify what that particular ingredient's purpose is in that formula. Once one knows that, one can go to that section in a *materia medica* or *ben cao* and choose another ingredient with the same or closely similar flavor, nature, functions, and indications. Thus one should not become unduly upset if one wishes to use one of the formulas in this book and a single medicinal is not available. Simply substitute or just leave it out unless it is the ruling ingredient in the formula. If it is the ruling ingredient in the formula, the ingredient that the rest of the formula is crafted around, and it is not available, then pick another formula whose functions, indications, and ingredients are basically analogous. Usually one will find a number of formulas in each section which are only variations on a single theme.

Where to Find Out More Information on Individual Chinese Medicinals

When prescribing a Chinese medicinal wine, as when prescribing any Chinese herbal formula, one should know what the purpose and functions of each ingredient in the formula are before prescribing that formula. Only in possession of this knowledge can one be sure a given formula fits a specific patient. If one wants to find out more information on any of the individual medicinals comprising the formulas in this book, most of these are discussed in Bensky and Gamble's *Chinese Herbal Medicine: Materia Medica* published by Eastland Press, Seattle, WA. Those that are not included in that standard text will typically be found in Hong-yen Hsu's *Oriental Materia Medica: A Concise Guide* published by the Oriental Healing Arts Institute, Long Beach, CA.

Tiger Bone

Os Tigridis (*Hu Gu*) or Tiger Bone is an ingredient in a number of Chinese medicinal wine formulas. These appear under the categories of strengthening the sinews and bones, dispelling wind, and formulas for traumatic injuries. As the reader hopefully is aware, tigers are an endangered species partly because of their use in Chinese medicine. Many people say that what is actually used in place of Tiger Bone in formulas containing that ingredient is pig bone, that there just are not enough tigers available for their bones to be used in so many Chinese patent medicines. Even if that is true, calling this ingredient Tiger Bone only continues to make the real thing a sought after and precious commodity. Thus calling this ingredient Tiger Bone does contribute to the tiger's extinction even if pig bone is used in most patent medicines listing this ingredient.

Because of this, I have chosen not to include any formulas whose name contains the words Tiger Bone or in which Tiger Bone is the main ingredient. In my research, this amounted to some 20 medicinal wines listed by various Chinese sources, both premodern and contemporary. In several other formulas, Tiger Bone is just one of a large number of ingredients. In my opinion, this ingredient is not absolutely essential, and so I have deleted it from these formulas. This only amounts to three or four in the entire book.

Western science has shown that the body does metabolize bone matrix calcium differently than calcium from limestone and shells. Calcium from bone matrix can help build strong bones and increase bone density. Therefore, patients wishing to build stronger bones and using formulas from the bone and sinew strengthening category should consider taking bone matrix calcium which is available at health food stores. It is also possible to add pig or some other type of animal bones to the wines designed for this purpose.

4

Supplementing Vacuity Detriment

The wines in this chapter all supplement and boost vacuity and detriment, deficiency and debility. These vacuities and deficiencies include those of the qi and blood, yin and yang. Such vacuities may be due to constitutional weakness, aging, overtaxation, bedroom or sexual taxation, prolonged disease, or the aftermath of a severe disease. In TCM, there are four basic types of vacuity, each with their own signs and symptoms. These are qi vacuity, blood vacuity, yin vacuity, and yang vacuity. There are wines and tinctures in this chapter to supplement each of these individually and combinations of these simultaneously.

In particular, many of the wines in this chapter supplement both the liver and kidneys. This means that they supplement liver blood and kidney yin and/or yang. Since liver blood is closely associated with the essence, the blood and essence sharing a common source, such formulas also increase, boost, or fill the essence. Most of the symptoms of aging have to do first with qi and yin vacuity and then with concomitant yang vacuity. This manifests as low back soreness and weakness, decline in reproductive function and ability, diminished hearing and vision, greying of the hair, etc. These symptoms are mostly associated in TCM with liver and kidney dual vacuity.

In China, therefore, these tinctures are generally used by the elderly, meaning those over 60 years of age. They are also used more often in the winter than the summer. The elderly are, by definition, vacuous. Therefore, in order to restore balance and promote health, this vacuity should be supplemented. In those without clinical signs and symptoms of vacuity, unwarranted supplementation may actually cause disease. Traditional Chinese Medicine cures disease and promotes health by restoring balance. Excess qi, blood, yin, or yang which is not smoothly and harmoniously circulated, consumed, and transformed will only accumulate and be transmuted into some form of evil or disease-causing qi.

Therefore, these supplementing wines and tinctures should not be used recklessly by the young and fit. This may very well cause disease. Hence it is always advisable to get a professional diagnosis from a qualified TCM practitioner before taking any of these supplementing wines.

Zhong Zi Yao Jiu ([Boosting] Seed Medicinal Wine)

Functions: Engenders reproductive essence, regulates the menses, protects the origin

Mainly treats: Male and female infertility

Ingredients: Sclerotium Poriae Cocos (*Fu Ling*), 100g, Fructus Zizyphi Jujubae (*Da Zao*), 50g, Semen Juglandis Regiae (*Hu Tao Ren*), 36g, Radix Astragali Membranacei (*Huang Qi*), 6g, Radix Codonopsis Pilosulae (*Dang Shen*), 6g, Rhizoma Atractylodis Macrocephalae (*Bai Zhu*), 6g, Rhizoma Ligustici Wallichii (*Chuan Xiong*), 6g, stir-fried Radix Albus Paeoniae Lactiflorae (*Bai Shao*), 6g, Radix Rehmanniae (*Sheng Di*), 6g, prepared Radix Rehmanniae (*Shu Di*), 6g, Fructus Foeniculi Vulgaris (*Xiao Hui Xiang*), 6g, Fructus Rubi (*Fu Pen Zi*), 6g, Pericarpium Citri Reticulatae (*Chen Pi*), 6g, Lignum Aquilariae Agallochae (*Chen Xiang*), 6g, Radix Saussureae Seu Vladimiriae (*Mu Xiang*), 6g, Fructus Lycii Chinensis (*Gou Qi Zi*), 6g, Cortex Cinnamomi (*Rou Gui*), 6g, Fructus Amomi (*Sha Ren*), 6g, Gummum Olibani (*Ru Xiang*), 6g, Myrrha (*Mo Yao*), 6g, Fructus

Schizandrae Chinensis (*Wu Wei Zi*), 6g, Radix Glycyrrhizae (*Gan Cao*), 6g

Method of preparation: Place the above medicinals in a large jar and add 600g of Honey, 2kg of white alcohol, and 1kg of rice wine. Allow to tincture for 15 days.

Method of administration: Take 30ml each time, 2 times per day.

Huang Qi Jiu (Astragalus Wine)

Functions: Boosts the qi, stimulates the engenderment and transformation of blood, stops vacuity sweating

Mainly treats: Qi vacuity, vacuity sweating, spleen/stomach vacuity weakness, diminished appetite and torpid intake, heart palpitation, shortness of breath, lack of strength in the four extremities, qi vacuity rectal prolapse

Ingredients: Radix Astragali Membranacei (*Huang Qi*), 300g

Method of preparation: Place the above medicinal in a large jar and soak in 2 qts. of alcohol. Seal the lid and allow to tincture for 1 month. Open, remove the dregs, and store for use.

Method of administration: Take 10-60cc 3 times per day.

Hu Tao Jiu (Walnut Wine)

Functions: Supplements the lungs and kidneys, boosts the essence, transforms phlegm, stops coughing, moistens the muscles and skin

Mainly treats: Kidney vacuity low back aching and pain, coarse, rough skin and muscles

Ingredients: Semen Juglandis Regiae (*Hu Tao Ren*), 300g

Method of preparation: Crush the above ingredient in a pestle and place in a large jar. Soak in 1 qt. alcohol for 1 month and seal the lid. Open, remove the dregs, and decant.

Method of administration: Take 60cc 3 times per day.

Hong Zao Jiu (Red Date Wine)

Functions: Supplements the qi and fortifies the spleen, nourishes the blood and promotes digestion

Mainly treats: Minor spleen qi vacuity and indigestion due to stomach weakness

Ingredients: Fructus Zizyphi Jujubae (*Da Zao*), 600g

Method of preparation: Place the above medicinal in a large jar and soak in 1 qt. of alcohol for 1 month. Seal the lid. Later, open, remove the dregs, and store for use.

Method of administration: Take 10-40cc 3 times per day.

Du Zhong Jiu (Eucommia Wine)

Functions: Supports the righteous, supplements the essence, and boosts the kidneys

Mainly treats: Kidney vacuity low back and knee soreness and weakness

Ingredients: Cortex Eucommiae Ulmoidis (*Du Zhong*), 300g

Method of preparation: Place the above medicinal in 2 qts. alcohol and soak for 1 month. Seal the lid. Later, open, remove the dregs, and store for use.

Method of administration: Take 10-60cc 3 times per day.

Tu Si Zi Jiu (Cuscuta Wine)

Functions: Supplements the kidneys and assists the life gate fire, stops vacuity diarrhea

Mainly treats: Kidney vacuity low back pain, life gate fire debility and weakness, cock-crow diarrhea

Ingredients: Semen Cuscutae (*Tu Si Zi*), 300g

Method of preparation: Place the above ingredient in a large jar and soak in 2 qts. alcohol for 2 months. Seal the lid. Later, open, remove the dregs, and decant.

Method of administration: Take 10-40cc 3 times per day.

Mai Men Dong Jiu (Ophiopogon Wine)

Functions: Supplements the kidneys, heart, lungs, and brain, stops cough and levels wheezing, clears heart fire

Mainly treats: Palpitations, restlessness, and insomnia due to heart vacuity, lung yin vacuity cough and asthma

Ingredients: Tuber Ophiopogonis Japonicae (*Mai Men Dong*), 300g

Method of preparation: Place the above ingredient in a large jar and soak in 2 qts. alcohol for 1 month. Seal the lid. Later, open, remove the dregs, and store for use.

Method of administration: Take 10-60cc 3 times per day.

Gou Qi Zi Jiu (Lycium Wine)

Functions: Enriches the kidneys and nourishes the liver, brightens the eyes

Mainly treats: Night blindness and blurred vision, foot and knee atony and weakness, upper back aching and pain, prolonged accumulation of wind toxins with the body, women's postpartum dizziness and vertigo

Ingredients: Fructus Lycii Chinensis (*Gou Qi Zi*), 300g

Method of preparation: Place the above medicinal in a large jar and soak in 2 qts alcohol for 2 months. Seal the lid. Later, open the lid, remove the dregs, and store for use.

Method of administration: Take 1-2 oz. before or after meals.

He Shou Wu Jiu (Polygonum Multiflorum Wine)

Functions: Supplements the kidneys and nourishes the liver, boosts the essence and blackens the hair, quiets the spirit

Mainly treats: Low back and knee soreness and weakness, blurred vision, premature greying of the hair, insomnia

Ingredients: Radix Polygoni Multiflori (*He Shou Wu*), 300g

Method of preparation: Place the above medicinal in a large jar and soak in 2 qts. of alcohol for 1 month. Seal the lid. Later, open, remove the dregs, and store for use.

Method of administration: Take 1-2 oz. before or after dinner.

Dang Gui Jiu (*Dang Gui* Wine)

Functions: Nourishes the blood, quickens the blood, regulates the menses

Mainly treats: Blood vacuity, blood stasis, and menstrual irregularity

Ingredients: Radix Angelicae Sinensis (*Dang Gui*), 300g

Method of preparation: Place the above medicinal in a large jar and soak in 2 qts. alcohol for 1 month. Seal the lid. Later, open, remove the dregs, and decant.

Method of administration: Take 10-60cc 3 times per day.

Shan Yao Jiu (Dioscorea Wine)

Functions: Supplements the spleen and kidneys, stops leakage

Mainly treats: Spleen/kidney vacuity diarrhea, spermatorrhea, polyuria, urinary incontinence, nocturia, and vacuity sweating

Ingredients: Radix Dioscoreae Oppositae (*Shan Yao*), 300g

Method of preparation: Place the above ingredient in a large jar and soak in 2 qts. of alcohol for 1 month. Seal the lid. Later, open, remove the dregs, and decant.

Method of administration: Take 10-40cc 3 times per day.

Method of modification: Add lemon juice to stop vacuity sweating and other symptoms of slippage.

Ren Shen Jiu (Ginseng Wine)

Functions: Supplements the original qi, supplements the lungs and fortifies the spleen, generates fluids, boosts the heart qi, and quiets the spirit

Mainly treats: Qi vacuity, shortness of breath, bodily fatigue, lack of strength, lack of appetite, loose stools, palpitations, insomnia, poor memory, dizziness, bodily vacuity in the aftermath of disease

Ingredients: Radix Panacis Ginseng (*Ren Shen*), 300g

Method of preparation: Place the above medicinal in a large jar and soak in 2 qts. of alcohol for 1 month. Seal the lid. Later, open and use. Typically, the Ginseng is left in the bottle or jar. When the first batch of wine is used, one can refill and repeat the process. The resulting tincture will be weaker but will have the same general effects, only milder.

Zhi Wu Jia Jiu (Siberian Ginseng Wine)

Functions: Boosts the qi and fortifies the spleen

Mainly treats: Qi vacuity, lack of strength, reduced appetite, loose stools

Ingredients: Radicis Eleutherococci Senticosi (*Zhi Wu Jia*), 60g

Method of preparation: Soak the Siberian Ginseng in 1kg of alcohol for 1/2 month.

Method of administration: Take 15ml each time, 2 times per day.

Fu Ling Jiu (Poria Wine)

Functions: Fortifies the spleen and harmonizes the center, disinhibits dampness and promotes urination, calms the heart and quiets the spirit

Mainly treats: Bodily weakness in the aftermath of disease, generalized lack of strength, chronic diarrhea, chronic gastritis, etc.

Ingredients: Sclerotium Poriae Cocos (*Fu Ling*), 60g

Method of preparation: Grind the Poria into pieces and soak in 1kg of rice wine for 7 days.

Method of administration: Take 20ml each time, 2 times per day.

Pu Tao Jiu (Grape Wine)

Functions: Boosts the qi, warms the kidneys, and warms the low back

Mainly treats: Heart palpitations, excessive sweating, low back soreness, edema, inhibited urination

Ingredients: Dry Fructus Viticis Viniferae (*Gan Pu Tao, i.e.,* Raisins), 500g

Method of preparation: Soak the Raisins in 1kg of rice wine for 1/2 month.

Method of administration: Take 30ml each time, 2 times per day.

Chong Cao Jiu (Cordyceps Wine)

Functions: Supplements the kidneys and enriches the lungs

Mainly treats: Impotence, spermatorrhea, taxation coughing of phlegm and blood, failure to recover after the detriment of illness

Ingredients: Cordyceps Sinensis (*Dong Chong Xia Cao*), 20g

Method of preparation: Grind into pieces and soak in 1kg of white alcohol for 1/2 month.

Method of administration: Take 1 teacup each evening.

Hai Ma Jiu (Seahorse Wine)

Functions: Supplements the kidneys and strengthens yang, quickens the blood and stops pain

Mainly treats: Impotence, urinary incontinence, cough and wheezing, injury and damage due to fall and strike

Ingredients: Hippocampus (*Hai Ma*), 30g

Method of preparation: Grind the Seahorses into pieces and soak in 0.5kg of white alcohol for 7 days.

Method of administration: Take 15ml each time, 2 times per day.

Long Yan Jiu (Longan Wine)

Functions: Supplements the heart and nourishes the blood

Mainly treats: Excessive worry and anxiety, heart palpitations, insomnia

Ingredients: Arillus Euphoriae Longanae (*Long Yan Rou*), no amount specified

Method of preparation: Place some Longans in alcohol and soak for 100 days. Then remove the dregs and store for use.

Method of preparation: Take 1 small teacup per day.

Shen Gui Bu Xu Jiu (Ginseng & *Dang Gui* Supplement Vacuity Wine)

Functions: Supplements the qi and harmonizes the blood, regulates the spleen and stomach, restores good color to the cheeks

Mainly treats: Qi and blood dual vacuity, a yellow face and thin muscles, exhaustion and fatigue due to overtaxation, dullness of essence spirit, spleen vacuity, devitalized appetite

Ingredients: Radix Angelicae Sinensis (*Quan Dang Gui*), 26g, Rhizoma Ligustici Wallichii (*Chuan Xiong*), 10g, stir-fried Radix Albus Paeoniae Lactiflorae (*Chao Bai Shao*), 18g, raw Radix Rehmanniae (*Sheng Di*), 15g, Radix Panacis Ginseng (*Ren Shen*), 15g, Rhizoma Atractylodis Macrocephalae (*Bai Zhu*), 26g, Sclerotium Poriae Cocos (*Fu Ling*), 20g, mix-fried Radix Glycyrrhizae (*Zhi Gan Cao*), 15g, Cortex Radicis Acanthopanacis (*Wu Jia Pi*), 25g, Fructus Zizyphi Jujubae (*Da Zao*), 36g, Semen Juglandis Regiae (*Hu Tao Rou*), 36g

Method of preparation: Grind the above 11 medicinals into fine powder. Place in a large jar and soak in 3 *jin* of alcohol. Boil for 1 hour and then remove from the heat and allow to cool. Then seal the jar and bury in the earth for 5 days. Then unearth and 3-7 days later open and remove the dregs. Decant and store for use.

Method of administration: Drink 1-2 teacups warm each morning, noon, and night.

Bai Hua Ru Yi Han Chun Jiu (White Flower Wish-fulfilling, Heart's Content Spring Wine)

Functions: Boosts the kidneys and secures the essence, strengthens yang and stands up the atonic (or flaccid)

Mainly treats: Kidney yang insufficiency, impotence, urinary dribbling and dripping, male sterility due to yang weakness, female infertility due to yin debility

Ingredients: Lignum Aquilariae Agallochae (*Chen Xiang*), 30g, Flos Rosae Rugosae (*Mei Gui Hua*), 30g, Flos Rosae Polyanthae (*Qiang Wei Hua*), 30g, Flos Pruni (*Mei Hua*), Flos Pruni Persicae (*Tao Hua*), 30g, Flos Allii Tuberosi (*Jiu Cai Hua*), 30g, Semen Juglandis Regiae (*Hu Tao Rou*), 240g

Method of preparation: Place the above 7 medicinals in a large jar and soak in 2.5kg of rice wine and 2.5kg of white alcohol. Seal the lid. After 1 month, open, remove the dregs, and store for use.

Method of administration: Drink whatever amount one wishes.

Hong Yan Jiu (Red Cheeks Wine)

Functions: Supplements the kidneys and moistens dryness

Mainly treats: Kidney vacuity low back pain. Prolonged use reddens and moistens the facial complexion and strengthens and fortifies the elderly.

Ingredients: Semen Juglandis Regiae (*Hu Tao Ren*), 60g, small Fructus Zizyphi Jujubae (*Xiao Hong Zao*), 60g, Mel (*i.e.,* Honey, *Bai*

Mi), 60g, Semen Pruni Armeniacae (*Xing Ren*), 30g, Butter (*Su You*), 30g

Method of preparation: First melt the butter and honey together. Add this to 750g of alcohol. Then grind the Walnuts, Dates, and Apricot Seeds and add these to the alcohol. Seal the lid and soak for 21 days. Then open, remove the dregs, and store for use.

Method of administration: Take 15ml each time, 2 times per day.

Shan Yao Jiu (Dioscorea Wine)

Functions: Enriches lung & kidney yin, supplements vacuity, and astringes essence

Mainly treats: Lung/kidney yin deficiency, vacuity taxation phlegm cough, dry mouth, scanty fluids, night sweating, spermatorrhea

Ingredients: Radix Dioscoreae Oppositae (*Shan Yao*), 15g, Fructus Corni Officinalis (*Shan Zhu Yu*), 15g, Ganoderma (*Ling Zhi*), 15g

Method of preparation: Soak in 1kg of white alcohol for 1 month.

Method of administration: Take 10ml each time, 2 times per day.

Suan Zao Ren Jiu (Zizyphus Spinosa Wine)

Functions: Nourishes the five viscera, moistens the skin and muscles, treats foot qi

Mainly treats: Foot qi aching and pain, muscles and skin coarse and rough, heart spirit not calm

Ingredients: Semen Zizyphi Spinosae (*Suan Zao Ren*), 30g, Radix Astragali Membranacei (*Huang Qi*), 30g, Tuber Asparagi Cochinensis (*Tian Men Dong*), 20g, Sclerotium Rubrum Poriae Cocos (*Chi Fu Ling*), 30g, Radix Ledebouriellae Sesloidis (*Fang Feng*), 20g, Radix Angelicae Pubescentis (*Du Huo*), 20g, Semen Cannabis Sativae (*Huo Ma Ren*), 100g, Cortex Cinnamomi (*Rou Gui*), 20g, Cortex Radicis Acanthopanacis (*Wu Jia Pi*), Radix Achyranthis Bidentatae (*Niu Xi*), 50g, Pulvis Cornu Antelopis Saigae Tataricis (*Ling Yan Jiao Fen*), 6g, dry Fructus Viticis Viniciferae (*Gan Pu Tao, i.e.,* Raisins), 50g

Method of preparation: Pound the above 12 medicinals with a pestle to break them up. Then place them in a large jar and soak them in 3 *jin* of mellow wine. Seal the lid. Allow to tincture for 7 days and then open. Discard the dregs.

Method of administration: Drink warm before eating each morning, noon, and night whatever amount one wants.

Shen Zhu Jiu (Ginseng & Atractylodes Wine)

Functions: Boosts the qi and fortifies the spleen

Mainly treats: Spleen/stomach qi vacuity, shortness of breath, lack of strength, a yellow face and thin body, reduced food consumption, and loose stools

Ingredients: Radix Panacis Ginseng (*Ren Shen*), 20g, or Radix Codonopsis Pilosulae (*Dang Shen*), 30g, mix-fried Radix Glycyrrhizae (*Zhi Gan Cao*), 30g, Sclerotium Poriae Cocos (*Bai Fu Ling*), 40g, stir-fried Rhizoma Atractylodis Macrocephalae (*Chao Bai Zhu*), 40g, raw Rhizoma Zingiberis (*Sheng Jiang*), 20g, Fructus Zizyphi Jujubae (*Da Zao*), 30g

Method of preparation: Break up the above 6 medicinals in a mortar. Place in a large jar and soak in 2 *jin* of yellow wine (*i.e.*, rice wine or sake). Seal the lid. After allowing to tincture for 3 days, open, remove the dregs, and store for use.

Method of administration: Take 1-2 teacups warm on an empty stomach 1 time each morning and evening.

Method of modification: For more serious damp phlegm, add Rhizoma Pinelliae Ternatae (*Ban Xia*), 30g, and Pericarpium Citri Reticulatae (*Chen Pi*), 20g. If there is simultaneous vomiting, glomus and oppression, and pain in the stomach and epigastrium, add Radix Saussureae Seu Vladimiriae (*Mu Xiang*), 20g, and Fructus Amomi (*Sha Ren*), 25g.

Note: This is just the tincture form of *Si Jun Zi Tang* (Four Gentlemen Decoction).

Hai Xia Jiu (Shrimp Wine)

Functions: Supplements the kidneys and strengthens yang

Mainly treats: Kidney yang insufficiency, impotence, low back soreness, women's postpartum agalactia

Ingredients: Dry Shrimp (*Gan Hai Xia*), 12g, Semen Cuscutae (*Tu Si Zi*), 12g, Semen Juglandis Regiae (*Hu Tao Ren*), 6g, Cortex Eucommiae Ulmoidis (*Du Zhong*), 6g, stir-fried Radix Morindae Officinalis (*Ba Ji Tian*), 6g, Cinnabar (*Zhu Sha*), 6g, Fructus Psoraleae Corylifoliae (*Bu Gu Zhi*), 6g, Fructus Lycii Chinensis (*Gou Qi Zi*), 6g, Radix Dipsaci (*Xu Duan*), 6g, Radix Achyranthis Bidentatae (*Niu Xi*), 6g, Semen Gossypii Herbacei (*Mian Hua Zi Ren*), 6g

Method of preparation: Grind the above ingredients into pieces and soak in 1kg of alcohol for 15 days.

Method of administration: Take 9g each time, 2 times per day.

Note: Do not use this wine if there are any skin rashes. Shrimp are contraindicated in such cases because of their emitting nature.

Lu Rong Jiu (Deer Antler Wine)

Functions: Strengthens yang, strengthens the sinews

Mainly treats: Generalized vacuity and deficiency, weak sinews and bones, impotence, polyuria

Ingredients: Cornu Parvum Cervi (*Lu Rong*), 15g, Radix Dioscoreae Oppositae (*Shan Yao*), 30g

Method of preparation: Soak in 500g of white alcohol for 7 days.

Method of administration: Take 20ml each time, 2 times per day.

Ge Jie Jiu (Gecko Wine)

Functions: Supplements the lungs and boosts the kidneys, promotes the absorption of qi and stabilizes wheezing

Mainly treats: Vacuity taxation, exertional wheezing, cough, shortness of breath, impotence

Ingredients: Gecko (*Ge Jie*), 1 pair

Method of preparation: Remove the head, feet, and tail. Then cut into small pieces. Soak in 500g of yellow (*i.e.*, rice) wine for 7 days.

Method of administration: Take 30g each time, 2 times per day.

Tao Ren Zhu Sha Jiu (Persica & Cinnabar Wine)

Functions: Quickens the blood and quiets the spirit

Mainly treats: Cramping, aching, and pain in the vessels of the lateral costal region, a lusterless facial color, blood stasis, chest *bi*, heart palpitations

Ingredients: Semen Pruni Persicae (*Tao Ren*), 100g, Cinnabar (*Zhu Sha*), 10g

Method of preparation: Place the Persica in a large jar and soak in 1 *jin* of mellow wine. Seal the lid and cook. Then remove from the heat and allow to cool. Remove the dregs and add the finely ground Cinnabar and stir.

Method of administration: Take whenever necessary, 1-2 small cups each time warm.

Contraindications: Do not eat sheep's blood when using this remedy. This formula is not appropriate to be used by women.

E Jiao Jiu (Gelatinum Corii Asini Wine)

Functions: Supplements the blood and stops bleeding, enriches yin and moistens the lungs

Mainly treats: Yin vacuity cough, dizziness, heart palpitations, vacuity taxation, hemoptysis, hematemesis, *beng lou* or uterine bleeding

Ingredients: Gelatinum Corii Asini (*E Jiao*), 400g

Method of preparation: Cook the Gelatinum Corii Asini in 1 *jin* of alcohol over low heat until completely dissolved. Then add 2 *jin* more of alcohol and continue cooking. Allow to cool to warm before taking.

Method of administration: Divide this amount into 4 portions. Drink a little bit on an empty stomach. There is no restriction as to when one can take this. If one has not healed by the time one has finished this amount, prepare a second batch as above and take again.

Contraindications: Do not use this formula if suffering from spleen/stomach vacuity weakness, diarrhea and vomiting, or indigestion.

Ji Xue Teng Jiu (Millettia Wine)

Functions: Supplements the blood and quickens the blood, soothes the sinews and opens the network vessels

Mainly treats: Unsoothed sinew and bone aching and pain, low back and knee chilly pain, detriment and damage due to falling and striking, wind, cold, damp *bi*, vacuity detriment of the sinews due to twisting, numbness of the hands and feet, women's irregular menstruation

Ingredients: Caulis Millettiae Seu Spatholobi (*Ji Xue Teng*), 400g

Method of preparation: Place the above medicinal in a large jar and soak in 2 *jin* of mellow wine. Seal the lid. Seven days later open, remove the dregs, and store for use.

Method of administration: Take 1-2 teacups morning and evening warm on an empty stomach.

Nu Zhen Zi Jiu (Ligustrum Lucidum Wine)

Functions: Supplements the kidneys and enriches yin, nourishes the liver and brightens the eyes

Mainly treats: Yin vacuity, internal heat, low back and knee soreness and weakness, dizziness and vertigo, premature greying of the hair

Ingredients: Fructus Ligustri Lucidi (*Nu Zhen Zi*), 250g

Method of preparation: In a mortar and pestle, break up the above medicinal and then place in a large jar. Soak in 1.5 *jin* of mellow wine. Seal the lid. Then open after 5 days, remove the dregs, and store for use.

Method of administration: Take 1-2 teacups in the morning and evening warm on an empty stomach.

Lu Rong Jiu (Cornu Parvum Cervi Wine)

Functions: Supplements kidney yang, boosts the essence and blood, strengthens the sinews and bones

Mainly treats: Male vacuity taxation essence debility, dual deficiency of essence and blood, impotence, low back and knee soreness and pain, fear of cold, lack of strength, bones weak, fatigued spirit, urinary incontinence, spermatorrhea, dizziness, tinnitus, poor growth in children, female infertility, uterine bleeding, and abnormal vaginal discharge when due to vacuity cold

Ingredients: Cornu Parvum Cervi (*Lu Rong*), 10g, Radix Dioscoreae Oppositae (*Shan Yao*), 30g

Method of preparation: Place the above medicinals in a large jar and soak in 1 *jin* of mellow wine. Seal the lid. Open 7 days later, remove the dregs, and store for use.

Method of administration: Drink 1-2 small teacups 3 times per day on an empty stomach.

Xi Yang Shen Jiu (American Ginseng Wine)

Functions: Supplements the qi and nourishes yin, clears fire and generates fluids

Mainly treats: Yin vacuity, fire effulgence, cough with phlegm and blood, heat diseases which have damaged both qi and yin, vexation, fatigue, a thirsty mouth, fluid and humor insufficiency, a dry mouth and parched throat

Ingredients: Radix Panacis Qinquefolii (*Xi Yang Shen*), 30g

Method of preparation: Place the above medicinal in a large jar and soak in 1 *jin* of rice wine. After 7 days, open and the formula is ready for use.

Method of administration: Take 1 small teacup 2 times per day on an empty stomach.

Contraindications: Do not use in case of central yang debility and deficiency or if the stomach is cold and damp.

Ming Mu Jiu (Eye-brightening Wine)

Functions: Nourishes liver blood and brightens the eyes, enriches the kidneys and boosts the marrow

Mainly treats: Impotence, spermatorrhea, low back and knee soreness and weakness, dizziness, vertigo, tearing eyes on exposure to wind, blurred vision

Ingredients: Fructus Lycii Chinensis (*Gou Qi Zi*), 80g

Method of preparation: Smash in a mortar and pestle and place in a large jar. Soak in ½ *jin* of mellow wine and seal the lid. After 7 days, open and remove the dregs. Store for use.

Method of administration: Drink 1-2 teacups per time, but do not overindulge

Gou Qi Sheng Di Jiu (Lycium & Rehmannia Wine)

Functions: Supplements the essence and boosts the kidneys, enriches yin, nourishes the liver, and brightens the eyes

Mainly treats: Impotence, spermatorrhea, vexatious heat, dizziness, low back and knee soreness and weakness, blurred vision

Ingredients: Fructus Lycii Chinensis (*Gou Qi Zi*), 250g, raw Radix Rehmanniae (*Sheng Di*), 300g

Method of preparation: Pestle the above two medicinals and place in a large jar. Soak in 3 *jin* of alcohol and seal the lid. Open the lid after 15 days, remove the dregs, and store for use.

Method of administration: Take 10-20ml warm on an empty stomach 1 time morning and evening.

Contraindications: Do not eat turnips, onions, or scallions.

Yi Shou Jiu (Boosting Longevity Wine)

Functions: Supplements the qi and blood, strengthens the essence spirit, moistens the muscles and skin, promotes the appetite, long term use boosts longevity

Mainly treats: Qi and blood insufficiency, yellow facial color, muscular thinness, low back soreness, tired feet, impotence, spermatorrhea, excessive dreams, easy fright, heart spirit absentminded, palpitations, poor memory

Ingredients: Raw Radix Rehmanniae (*Sheng Di*), 40g, prepared Radix Rehmanniae (*Shu Di*), 40g, Tuber Asparagi Cochinensis (*Tian Men Dong*), 40g, Tuber Ophiopogonis Japonicae (*Mai Men Dong*), 40g, Radix Angelicae Sinensis (*Dang Gui*), 40g, Radix Achyranthis Bidentatae (*Niu Xi*), 40g, Cortex Eucommiae Ulmoidis (*Du Zhong*), 40g, Fructus Foeniculi Vulgaris (*Xiao Hui Xiang*), 40g, Radix Morindae Officinalis (*Ba Ji Tian*), 40g, Rhizoma Ligustici Wallichii (*Chuan Xiong*), 40g, Radix Albus Paeoniae Lactiflorae (*Bai Shao*), 40g, Sclerotium Poriae Cocos (*Bai Fu Ling*), 40g, Rhizoma Anemarrhenae (*Zhi Mu*), 40g, Fructus Amomi (*Sha Ren*), 24g, Rhizoma Atractylodis Macrocephalae (*Bai Zhu*), 24g, Radix Polygalae Tenuifoliae (*Yuan Zhi*), 24g, Fructus Psoraleae Corylifoliae (*Bu Gu Zhi*), 24g, Radix Saussureae Seu Vladimiriae (*Mu Xiang*), 12g, Radix

53

Panacis Ginseng (*Ren Shen*), 12g, Rhizoma Acori Graminei (*Shi Chang Pu*), 12g, Semen Biotae Orientalis (*Bai Zi Ren*), 12g, Cortex Phellodendri (*Huang Bai*), 50g, Fructus Lycii Chinensis (*Gou Qi Zi*), 50g, Herba Cistanchis (*Rou Cong Rong*), 40g

Method of preparation: Pestle the above 24 medicinals and then place them in a large jar. Soak in 7 *jin* of yellow wine (*i.e.*, rice wine). Bring to a boil 100 times. Then seal the lid and bury in the earth for 3 days. This removes the fire toxins. Later remove the dregs and store for use.

Method of administration: Drink whatever amount one wishes per day, remembering that this is a medicine—not a beverage.

Gu Ti Di Huang Jiu (Securing the Body Rehmannia Wine)

Functions: Supplements vacuity and blackens the hair, restores color to the cheeks

Mainly treats: Yin and yang dual vacuity, qi weakness and essence deficiency, premature aging and debility

Ingredients: Raw Radix Rehmanniae (*Sheng Di*), 30g, prepared Radix Rehmanniae (*Shu Di*), 30g, Tuber Asparagi Cochinensis (*Tian Men Dong*), 30g, Tuber Ophiopogonis Japonicae (*Mai Men Dong*), 30g, Sclerotium Poriae Cocos (*Bai Fu Ling*), 30g, Radix Panacis Ginseng (*Ren Shen*), 30g

Method of preparation: Pestle the above 6 medicinals and place in a large jar. Soak for 3 days in 2 *jin* of alcohol. Then boil over a fire until the wine turns black. Remove the dregs and store for use.

Method of administration: Take on an empty stomach whatever amount one wishes at no fixed times.

Er Dong Er Di Jiu (Two Dong & Two Di Wine)

Functions: Supplements the kidneys and increases the essence, quiets the spirit and stabilizes the orientation (*i.e.*, the emotions or affect)

Mainly treats: Kidney vacuity, essence deficiency, middle-aged impotence, blurred vision in the elderly, spirit orientation absentmindedness, low back and knee soreness and weakness

Ingredients: Semen Cuscutae (*Tu Si Zi*), 120g, Herba Cistanchis (*Rou Cong Rong*), Tuber Asparagi Cochinensis (*Tian Men Dong*), 60g, raw Radix Rehmanniae (*Sheng Di*), 60g, prepared Radix Rehmanniae (*Shu Di*), 60g, Radix Dioscoreae Oppositae (*Shan Yao*), 60g, Radix Achyranthis Bidentatae (*Niu Xi*), 60g, Cortex Eucommiae Ulmoidis (*Du Zhong*), 60g, Radix Morindae Officinalis (*Ba Ji Tian*), 60g, Fructus Lycii Chinensis (*Gou Qi Zi*), 60g, Fructus Corni Officinalis (*Shan Zhu Yu*), 60g, Radix Panacis Ginseng (*Ren Shen*), 60g, Sclerotium Poriae Cocos (*Bai Fu Ling*), 60g, Fructus Schizandrae Chinensis (*Wu Wei Zi*), 60g, Radix Saussureae Seu Vladimiriae (*Mu Xiang*), 60g, Semen Biotae Orientalis (*Bai Zi Ren*), 60g, Fructus Rubi (*Fu Pen Zi*), 45g, Semen Plantaginis (*Che Qian Zi*), 45g, Cortex Radicis Lycii (*Di Gu Pi*), 45g, Rhizoma Acori Graminei (*Shi Chang Pu*), 30g, Fructus Zanthoxyli Bungeani (*Chuan Jiao*), 30g, Radix Polygalae Tenuifoliae (*Yuan Zhi*), 30g, Rhizoma Alismatis (*Ze Xie*), 30g

Method of preparation: Pestle the above 24 ingredients and place in a large jar. Soak in 6 *jin* of alcohol for 7-12 days. Then open and remove the dregs. Store for use.

55

Method of administration: Take 1 small teacup on an empty stomach morning and evening.

Que Lao Jiu (Step Back from Old Age Wine)

Functions: Supplements the five viscera, fills the essence and marrow, blackens the hair, moistens the muscles and skin, recedes old age and rolls back the years

Mainly treats: Essence and blood insufficiency, body debilitated and weak, loss of luster of the color of the cheeks, thinning hair

Ingredients: Flos Chrysanthemi Morifolii (*Gan Ju Hua*), 60g, Tuber Ophiopogonis Japonicae (*Mai Men Dong*), 60g, Fructus Lycii Chinensis (*Gou Qi Zi*), 60g, baked Rhizoma Atractylodis Macrocephalae (*Jiao Bai Zhu*), 60g, Rhizoma Acori Graminei (*Shi Chang Pu*), 60g, Radix Polygalae Tenuifoliae (*Yuan Zhi*), 60g, Sclerotium Poriae Cocos (*Fu Ling*), 70g, prepared Radix Rehmanniae (*Shu Di*), 60g, Radix Panacis Ginseng (*Ren Shen*), 30g, Cortex Cinnamomi (*Rou Gui*), 25g, Radix Polygoni Multiflori (*He Shou Wu*), 50g

Method of preparation: Pestle the above 11 medicinals and place in a large jar. Soak in 4 *jin* of mellow wine and seal the lid. After 5 days in the spring or summer and 7 days in the fall and winter, open and remove the dregs. Then store for use.

Method of administration: Take 1 small teacup warm before meals each day.

Shen Qi Jiu (Ginseng & Lycium Wine)

Functions: Boosts the essence and secures the marrow, enriches yin and brightens the eyes, moistens the five viscera, prolonged administration rolls back the years

Mainly treats: Kidney vacuity, essence deficiency, yang impotence, inability to achieve an erection, tinnitus, vertigo, a lusterless facial color

Ingredients: Fructus Lycii Chinensis (*Gou Qi Zi*), 30g, Radix Rehmanniae (*Di Huang*), 30g, Tuber Ophiopogonis Japonicae (*Mai Men Dong*), 18g, Semen Pruni Armeniacae (*Xing Ren*), 10g, Radix Panacis Ginseng (*Ren Shen*), 6g, Sclerotium Poriae Cocos (*Fu Ling*), 10g

Method of preparation: Pestle the above 6 ingredients and place in a large jar. Soak in 2 *jin* of alcohol and seal the lid. Open after 7 days, remove the dregs, and store for use.

Method of administration: Take 10ml warm before meals 1 time in the morning and evening.

Shen Shu Jiu (Ginseng & Zanthoxylum Wine)

Functions: Supplements the qi and harmonizes the center, boosts the kidneys and quiets the heart

Mainly treats: Spleen/kidney yang vacuity, vacuity chill of the lower origin, dizziness and blurred vision, an ashen white facial color

Ingredients: Cinnabar (*Dan Sha*), 20g, Sclerotium Poriae Cocos (*Fu Ling*), 30g, Radix Panacis Ginseng (*Ren Shen*), 30g, Fructus Zantho-xyli Bungeani (*Shu Jiao*), 120g

Method of preparation: Grind the last 3 ingredients into a fine powder. Then place this and the Cinnabar into a large jar. Soak in 2 *jin* of mellow wine. Allow to tincture for 5 days in the spring and summer and for 7 days in the fall and winter. Remove the dregs and store for use.

Method of administration: Take 1 small teacup warm on an empty stomach before meals.

Bu Qi Yang Xue Jiu (Supplement the Qi, Nourish the Blood Wine)

Functions: Supplements the qi and blood, nourishes the heart and kidneys, fortifies the spleen and stomach, boosts the aged

Mainly treats: Qi and blood insufficiency, spleen/stomach vacuity weakness, palpitations, poor memory, vertigo and blurred vision

Ingredients: Fructus Psoraleae Corylifoliae (*Bu Gu Zhi*), 30g, prepared Radix Rehmanniae (*Shu Di*), 30g, raw Radix Rehmanniae (*Sheng Di*), 30g, Tuber Asparagi Cochinensis (*Tian Men Dong*), 30g, Tuber Ophiopogonis Japonicae (*Mai Men Dong*), 30g, Radix Panacis Ginseng (*Ren Shen*), 30g, Radix Angelicae Sinensis (*Dang Gui*), 30g, Rhizoma Ligustici Wallichii (*Chuan Xiong*), 30g, Radix Albus Paeoniae Lactiflorae (*Bai Shao*), 30g, Sclerotium Poriae Cocos (*Fu Ling*), 30g, Semen Biotae Orientalis (*Bai Zi Ren*), 30g, Fructus Amomi (*Sha Ren*), 30g, Rhizoma Acori Graminei (*Shi Chang Pu*), 30g, Radix Polygalae Tenuifoliae (*Yuan Zhi*), 30g, Radix Saussureae Seu Vladimiriae (*Mu Xiang*), 15g

Method of preparation: Pestle the above 15 medicinals and place in a large jar. Soak in 4 *jin* of alcohol. Then place over a fire and boil. Remove the dregs, allow to cool, and store for use.

Method of administration: Take 10-20ml warm each time at no fixed schedule.

Ren Shen Fu Ling Jiu (Ginseng & Poria Wine)

Functions: Supplements the qi and blood, boosts the spleen and stomach, loosens the diaphragm and promotes digestion

Mainly treats: Qi and blood deficiency and debility, spleen vacuity, stomach weakness, emaciated body, a sallow yellow facial color

Ingredients: Radix Panacis Ginseng (*Ren Shen*), 30g, raw Radix Rehmanniae (*Sheng Di*), 30g, Sclerotium Poriae Cocos (*Fu Ling*), 30g, Rhizoma Atractylodis Macrocephalae (*Bai Zhu*), 30g, Radix Albus Paeoniae Lactiflorae (*Bai Shao*), 30g, Radix Angelicae Sinensis (*Dang Gui*), 30g, Massa Medica Fermentata (*Hong Qu Mian*), Rhizoma Ligustici Wallichii (*Chuan Xiong*), 15g, Cortex Cinnamomi (*Rou Gui*), 120g

Method of preparation: Grind the above 9 ingredients into a fine powder and place in a large jar. Soak in *gao liang* wine (a type of sorghum wine with a very high alcohol content) for 4-5 days. Remove the dregs and add 250g of sugar.

Method of administration: Drink a small amount each day.

Zhou Gong Bai Sui Jiu (Master Zhou's Hundred Years Wine)

Functions: Strengthens the original qi, harmonizes the blood vessels, increases the essence, and supplements the brain

Mainly treats: Timid qi and fatigued spirit, body emaciated, low back soreness and weakness, palpitations, poor memory

Ingredients: Radix Astragali Membranacei (*Huang Qi*), 30g, Sclerotium Pararadicis Poriae Cocos (*Fu Shen*), 30g, Cortex Cinnamomi (*Rou Gui*), 10g, Radix Angelicae Sinensis (*Quan Dang Gui*), 18g, raw Radix Rehmanniae (*Sheng Di*), 20g, prepared Radix Rehmanniae (*Shu Di*), 20g, Radix Codonopsis Pilosulae (*Dang Shen*), 15g, Rhizoma Atractylodis Macrocephalae (*Bai Zhu*), 15g, Tuber Ophiopogonis Japonicae (*Mai Men Dong*), 15g, Sclerotium Poriae Cocos (*Fu Ling*), 15g, Pericarpium Citri Reticulatae (*Chen Pi*), 15g, Fructus Corni Officinalis (*Shan Zhu Yu*), 15g, Fructus Lycii Chinensis (*Gou Qi Zi*), 15g, Rhizoma Ligustici Wallichii (*Chuan Xiong*), 15g, Radix Ledebouriellae Sesloidis (*Fang Feng*), 15g, Colla Plastri Testudinis (*Gui Ban Jiao*), 15g, Fructus Schizandrae Chinensis (*Wu Wei Zi*), 12g, Radix Et Rhizoma Notopterygii (*Qiang Huo*), 12g

Method of preparation: Grind the above 18 medicinals into a fine powder. Place in a large jar and soak in 3 *jin* of *gao liang* wine. Open after 7 days, remove the dregs, and store for use.

Method of administration: Take 1 small teacup 3 times per day warm on an empty stomach.

Yang Rong Jiu (Nourish the Constructive Wine)

Functions: Supplements vacuity detriment, strengthens the physical strength, moistens the muscles and skin; prolonged administration boosts longevity

Mainly treats: Bodily debility and weakness, bodily fatigue, lack of strength, body thin and pallid

Ingredients: Sclerotium Poriae Cocos (*Fu Ling*), 50g, Flos Chrysanthemi Morifolii (*Gan Ju Hua*), 50g, Rhizoma Acori Graminei (*Shi Chang Pu*), 50g, Tuber Asparagi Cochinensis (*Tian Men Dong*), 50g, Rhizoma Atractylodis Macrocephalae (*Bai Zhu*), 50g, raw Rhizoma Polygonati (*Sheng Huang Jing*), 50g, raw Radix Rehmanniae (*Sheng Di*), 50g, Radix Panacis Ginseng (*Ren Shen*), 30g, Cortex Cinnamomi (*Rou Gui*), 30g, Radix Achyranthis Bidentatae (*Niu Xi*), 30g

Method of preparation: Grind the above 10 medicinals into a fine powder and place in a large jar. Soak in 3 *jin* of mellow wine for 5 days in the spring and summer and for 7 days in the fall and winter. Open the lid, remove the dregs, and store for use.

Method of administration: Take 1 medium teacup 1 time morning and evening warm on an empty stomach.

Yan Shou Jiu (Extend Longevity Wine)

Functions: Nourishes the visceral blood; prolonged administration boosts longevity

Mainly treats: Bodily exhaustion, lack of strength, reduced appetite, dizziness and vertigo, inhibited low back and knees

61

Ingredients: Rhizoma Polygonati (*Huang Jing*), 30g, Rhizoma Atractylodis (*Cang Zhu*), 30g, Tuber Asparagi Cochinensis (*Tian Men Dong*), 20g, Folium Pini (*Song Ye, i.e.*, Pine Needles), 40g, Fructus Lycii Chinensis (*Gou Qi Zi*), 30g

Method of preparation: Grind the above 5 ingredients into a fine powder and place in a large jar. Soak in 3 *jin* of mellow wine for 7 days. Then remove the dregs and store for use.

Method of administration: Take 1-2 small teacups morning and evening warm on an empty stomach.

Kang Zhuang Jiu (Robust Health Wine)

Functions: Boosts the liver and kidneys, blackens the hair; prolonged administration by the elderly fortifies the body

Mainly treats: Liver/kidney insufficiency, premature greying of the hair, bodily fatigue, lack of strength, low back and knee weakness

Ingredients: Fructus Lycii Chinensis (*Gou Qi Zi*), 45g, stir-fried Massa Medica Fermentata (*Chao Chen Qu*), 45g, Flos Chrysanthemi Morifolii (*Gan Ju Hua*), 45g, prepared Radix Rehmanniae (*Shu Di*), 45g, Cortex Cinnamomi (*Rou Gui*), 45g, Herba Cistanchis (*Rou Cong Rong*), 36g

Method of preparation: Grind the above 6 ingredients into a fine powder and place in a large jar. Soak in 3 *jin* of mellow wine for 5 days in the spring and summer and 7 days in the fall and winter. After that, add 2 *jin* of cold water and store for use.

Method of administration: Take a small amount warm on an empty stomach at no fixed times.

62

Xu Guo Gong Xian Jiu (Master Xu Guo's Immortality Wine)

Functions: Supplements the heart and spleen, nourishes the blood and quiets the spirit

Mainly treats: Heart blood insufficiency, palpitations, insomnia, poor memory, body vacuity and weakness in the aged

Ingredients: Arillus Euphoriae Longanae (*Long Yan Rou*), 2 *jin*

Method of preparation: Place the Longans in a large jar and soak in 4 *jin* of mellow wine. Seal the lid. A half month later, decant for use.

Method of administration: Drink whatever amount one wishes morning and night.

Di Huang Nian Qing Jiu (Rehmannia & Lycopodium Wine)

Functions: Supplements the liver and kidneys, blackens the hair; prolonged use improves hearing and brightens the eyes

Mainly treats: Liver/kidney deficiency detriment, premature greying of the hair, premature aging, decreased eyesight

Ingredients: Prepared Radix Rehmanniae (*Shu Di*), 100g, Herba Lycopodii Cernui (*Wan Nian Qing*), 150g, black Fructus Mori (*Hei Sang Shen*), 120g, black Semen Sesami Indici (*Hei Zhi Ma*), 60g, Radix Dioscoreae Oppositae (*Shan Yao*), 200g, Semen Lyoniae (*Nan Zhu Zi*), 30g, Fructus Zanthoxyli Bungeani (*Hua Jiao*), 30g, Semen Gingkonis Bilobae (*Bai Guo*), 15g, Fructus Dipsaci (*Ju Sheng Zi*), 45g

Method of preparation: Grind the above 9 medicinals into a fine powder and place in a large jar. Soak in 4 *jin* of alcohol for 7 days. Open, remove the dregs, and store for use.

Method of administration: Take 1-2 teacups warm on an empty stomach 1 time each morning and evening.

Contraindications: Do not eat radishes while taking this medicinal wine.

Hong Yan Jiu (Red Cheeks Wine)

Functions: Supplements the kidneys, blackens the hair, moistens the lungs, moistens the muscles and skin, restores the color of the cheeks, boosts the qi and harmonizes the spleen

Mainly treats: Lung/kidney dual vacuity, low back pain, weak lower limbs, cough, wheezing, constipation in the elderly, prolonged diarrhea

Ingredients: Semen Juglandis Regiae (*Hu Tao Ren*), 120g, Fructus Zizyphi Jujubae (*Da Zao*), 120g, Semen Pruni Armeniacae (*Xing Ren*), 30g, Honey (*Bai Mi*), 100g, Butter (*Su You*), 70g

Method of preparation: First dissolve the honey and butter in 2 *jin* of heated alcohol. Then add the other 3 ingredients and soak for 7 days. After that, open, remove the dregs, and store for use.

Method of administration: Take 2-3 teacups on an empty stomach morning and night.

Bu Yi Jiu (Supplementing & Boosting Wine)

Functions: Supplements the liver and kidneys, fills the essence and blood, quiets the spirit and brightens the eyes

Mainly treats: Liver/kidney vacuity detriment, lower back and lower limb weakness, dizziness and vertigo, spirit orientation absentmindedness or abstraction

Ingredients: Herba Cistanchis (*Rou Cong Rong*), Semen Myristicae Fragrantis (*Rou Dou Kou*), 15g, Fructus Corni Officinalis (*Shan Zhu Yu*), 45g, Cinnabar (*Zhu Sha*), 10g

Method of preparation: Pestle the first 3 ingredients and then place all 4 medicinals in a large jar. Soak in 2 *jin* of alcohol and seal the lid. Open after 7 days, decoct, and store for use.

Method of administration: Take 1-2 small teacups warm on an empty stomach morning and evening.

Ju Qi Tiao Yuan Jiu (Chrysanthemum & Lycium Regulate the Origin Wine)

Functions: Regulates the original qi, brightens the ears and the eyes; prolonged administration strengthens the body

Mainly treats: Sinew and bone soreness and pain, vacuity chill of the lower origin

Ingredients: Flos Chrysanthemi Morifolii (*Gan Ju Hua*), 90g, Fructus Lycii Chinensis (*Gou Qi Zi*), 90g, Radix Morindae Officinalis (*Ba Ji Tian*), 90g, Herba Cistanchis (*Rou Cong Rong*), 90g

65

Method of preparation: Grind the above 4 medicinals into a fine powder and place in a large jar. Soak in 4 *jin* of alcohol and seal the lid. After 7 days, add 3 *jin* of cold water.

Method of administration: Take 1-2 small teacups warm on an empty stomach 1 time each morning and evening.

Shan Zhu Cong Rong Jiu (Dioscorea, Cornus & Cistanches Wine)

Functions: Supplements the liver and kidneys, warms the low back and knees, quiets the spirit and tranquilizes the orientation (*i.e.*, emotions), fills the essence and supplements the brain

Main indications: Liver/kidney deficiency detriment, dizziness, tinnitus, palpitations, poor memory, low back and lower limb weakness, lack of warmth in the body and extremities

Ingredients: Radix Dioscoreae Oppositae (*Shan Yao*), 25g, Herba Cistanchis (*Rou Cong Rong*), 60g, Fructus Schizandrae Chinensis (*Wu Wei Zi*), 35g, Cortex Eucommiae Ulmoidis (*Du Zhong*), 40g, Radix Cyathulae (*Chuan Niu Xi*), 30g, Semen Cuscutae (*Tu Si Zi*), 30g, Sclerotium Poriae Cocos (*Fu Ling*), 30g, Rhizoma Alismatis (*Ze Xie*), 30g, prepared Radix Rehmanniae (*Shu Di*), 30g, Fructus Corni Officinalis (*Shan Zhu Yu*), 30g, Radix Morindae Officinalis (*Ba Ji Tian*), 30g, Radix Polygalae Tenuifoliae (*Yuan Zhi*), 30g

Method of preparation: Pestle the above 12 ingredients and place them in a large jar. Soak in 4 *jin* of mellow wine and seal the lid. After 5 days in the spring and summer and 7 days in the fall and winter, open and remove the dregs. Then store for use.

66

Method of administration: Take 1-2 small teacups warm on an empty stomach 1 time each morning and evening.

Chu Shi Zhu Yang Jiu (Mulberry Reinforcing Yang Wine)

Functions: Warms kidney yang, strengthens the sinews and bones, warms the spleen and stomach

Mainly treats: Kidney yang vacuity detriment, impotence, spermator-rhea, spleen/stomach vacuity cold, a lusterless facial color

Ingredients: Fructus Mori (*Chu Shi Zi, i.e., Sang Shen*), 100g, Cornu Parvum Cervi (*Lu Rong*), 10g, Radix Praeparatus Aconiti Carmichaeli (*Zhi Fu Zi*), 60g, Radix Cyathulae (*Chuan Niu Xi*), 60g, Radix Morindae Officinalis (*Ba Ji Tian*), 60g, Herba Dendrobii (*Shi Hu*), blast-fried Rhizoma Zingiberis (*Pao Jiang*), 30g, Cortex Cinnamomi (*Rou Gui*), 30g, Fructus Zizyphi Jujubae (*Da Zao*), 60g

Method of preparation: Grind the above 9 ingredients into fine powder and place in a large jar. Soak in 4 *jin* of mellow wine and seal the lid. Open after 8 days and remove the dregs. Then store for use.

Method of administration: Take 10ml warm on an empty stomach 1 time each morning and evening.

Ba Ji Shu Di Jiu (Morinda & Prepared Rehmannia Wine)

Functions: Supplements the kidneys and strengthens yang, grows the muscles and flesh, restores the color to the cheeks

Mainly treats: Prolonged kidney yang vacuity, impotence, premature ejaculation, low back and knee soreness and weakness

67

Ingredients: Radix Morindae Officinalis (*Ba Ji Tian*), 60g, prepared Radix Rehmanniae (*Shu Di*), 45g, Fructus Lycii Chinensis (*Gou Qi Zi*), 30g, Radix Praeparatus Aconiti Carmichaeli (*Zhi Fu Zi*), 20g, Flos Chrysanthemi Morifolii (*Gan Ju Hua*), 60g, Fructus Zanthoxyli Bungeani (*Shu Jiao*), 30g

Method of preparation: Pestle the above 6 medicinals and place in a large jar. Soak in 3 *jin* of mellow wine and seal the lid. Open after 5 days, remove the dregs, and decant.

Method of administration: Take 1-2 small teacups warm on an empty stomach each morning and night.

Yi Shen Ming Mu Jiu (Boost the Kidneys, Brighten the Eyes Wine)

Functions: Boosts the kidneys and supplements the liver, nourishes the heart, improves the hearing and brightens the eyes, restores the color to the cheeks

Mainly treats: Liver/kidney vacuity detriment, tinnitus, vertigo, low back soreness and tired feet, fatigued spirit, decline in strength

Ingredients: Fructus Rubi (*Fu Pen Zi*), 50g, Radix Morindae Officinalis (*Ba Ji Tian*), 35g, Herba Cistanchis (*Rou Cong Rong*), 35g, Radix Polygalae Tenuifoliae (*Yuan Zhi*), 35g, Radix Cyathulae (*Chuan Niu Xi*), 35g, Fructus Schizandrae Chinensis (*Wu Wei Zi*), 35g, Radix Dipsaci (*Xu Duan*), 35g, Fructus Corni Officinalis (*Shan Zhu Yu*), 30g

Method of preparation: Grind the above 8 medicinals into fine powder and place in a large jar. Soak in 2 *jin* of mellow wine and seal the lid. Allow to tincture 5 days in the spring and summer and 7 days in the fall and winter. Then open, remove the dregs, and add 2 *jin* of cold water. Store for use.

Method of administration: Take 10-15ml warm on an empty stomach 1 time each morning and evening. Prolonged administration boosts the effectiveness of this formula.

Bu Jing Yi Lao Jiu (Supplement the Essence, Boost the Old Wine)

Functions: Supplements vacuity detriment, boosts the essence and blood; prolonged administration boosts the elderly

Mainly treats: Vacuity taxation detriment and damage, essence blood insufficiency, emaciated body, and ashen, old facial color, reduced appetite, kidney vacuity impotence, low back and knee soreness and weakness

Ingredients: Prepared Radix Rehmanniae (*Shu Di*), 120g, Radix Angelicae Sinensis (*Quan Dang Gui*), 150g, Rhizoma Ligustici Wallichii (*Chuan Xiong*), 45g, Cortex Eucommiae Ulmoidis (*Du Zhong*), 45g, Sclerotium Poriae Cocos (*Fu Ling*), 45g, Radix Glycyrrhizae (*Gan Cao*), 30g, Fructus Rosae Laevigatae (*Jin Ying Zi*), 30g, Herba Epimedii (*Yin Yang Huo*), 30g, Herba Dendrobii (*Jin Shi Hu*), 90g

Method preparation: Grind the above 9 ingredients into a fine powder and place in a large jar. Soak in 3 *jin* of alcohol and seal the lid. Allow to tincture 7 days in the spring and summer and 14 days in the fall and winter. Then open, remove the dregs, and store for use.

Method of administration: Take 1-2 teacups on an empty stomach 1 time each morning and evening.

69

Pi Shen Liang Zhu Jiu (Spleen/Kidney Dual Assisting Wine)

Functions: Increases the essence and supplements the marrow, fortifies spleen and nourishes the stomach; prolonged administration fortifies the physical body

Mainly treats: Spleen/kidney dual debility, male impotence, female menstrual irregularity, red and white abnormal vaginal discharge

Ingredients: Rhizoma Atractylodis Macrocephalae (*Bai Zhu*), 30g, Pericarpium Viridis Citri Reticulatae (*Qing Pi*), 30g, raw Radix Rehmanniae (*Sheng Di*), 30g, Cortex Magnoliae Officinalis (*Hou Po*), 30g, Cortex Eucommiae Ulmoidis (*Du Zhong*), 30g, Fructus Psoraleae Corylifoliae (*Bu Gu Zhi*), 30g, Pericarpium Citri Reticulatae (*Chen Pi*), 30g, Fructus Zanthoxyli Bungeani (*Chuan Jiao*), 30g, Sodium Chloride (*Qing Yan, i.e.,* salt), 15g, stir-fried Fructus Glycinis Hispidae (*Hei Dou, i.e.*, Black Soy Beans), 60g, Radix Morindae Officinalis (*Ba Ji Tian*), 30g, Sclerotium Poriae Cocos (*Fu Ling*), 30g, Fructus Foeniculi Vulgaris (*Xiao Hui Xiang*), 30g, Herba Cistanchis (*Rou Cong Rong*), 30g

Method of preparation: Grind the above 14 ingredients into a fine powder and place in a large jar. Soak in 3 *jin* of *gao liang* wine and seal the lid. Allow to tincture 7 days in the spring and summer and 10 days in the fall and winter. Open, remove the dregs, and store for use.

Method of administration: Take 1-2 teacups warm on an empty stomach each morning and evening.

Contraindications: Do not eat beef or horse meat while taking this formula. Pregnant women should also not take this wine.

Cong Rong Qiang Zhuang Jiu (Cistanches Strengthening Wine)

Functions: Supplements and boosts the liver and kidneys, improves the hearing and brightens the eyes, strengthens the sinews and bones; habitual administration fortifies the body and boosts longevity

Mainly treats: Liver/kidney vacuity detriment, aching and pain in the abdomen and lateral costal regions, chilly vacuity of the lower origin

Ingredients: Herba Cistanchis (*Rou Cong Rong*), 50g, Radix Cyathulae (*Chuan Niu Xi*), 40g, Semen Cuscutae (*Tu Si Zi*), Radix Praeparatus Aconiti Carmichaeli (*Zhi Fu Zi*), 20g, Fructus Zanthoxyli Bungeani (*Jiao Hong*), 30g, Semen Myristicae Fragrantis (*Rou Dou Kou Ren*), 20g, Fructus Psoraleae Corylifoliae (*Bu Gu Zhi*), 25g, Fructus Mori (*Sang Shen*), 25g, Radix Morindae Officinalis (*Ba Ji Tian*), 30g, Radix Saussureae Seu Vladimiriae (*Mu Xiang*), 15g, Cornu Parvum Cervi (*Lu Rong*), 10g, Cortex Cinnamomi (*Rou Gui*), 20g, Semen Cnidii Monnieri (*She Chuang Zi*), 15g, blast-fried Rhizoma Zingiberis (*Pao Jiang*), 20g

Method of preparation: Grind the above 14 medicinals into fine powder and place in a large jar. Soak in 3 *jin* of mellow wine and seal the lid. Allow to tincture for 5 days in the spring and summer and 7 days in the fall and winter. Then open, remove the dregs, and store for use.

Method of administration: Take 1-2 small teacups warm on an empty stomach 1 time each morning and evening.

Zhu Yang Jiu (Reinforce Yang Wine)

Functions: Supplements the kidneys and strengthens yang

Mainly treats: Impotence

Ingredients: Radix Codonopsis Pilosulae (*Dang Shen*), 15g, prepared Radix Rehmanniae (*Shu Di*), 15g, Fructus Lycii Chinensis (*Gou Qi Zi*), 15g, Semen Astragali (*Sha Yuan Ji Li*), 10g, Herba Epimedii (*Yin Yang Huo*), 10g, Flos Caryophylli (*Ding Xiang*), Radix Polygalae Tenuifoliae (*Yuan Zhi*), 4g, Lignum Aquilariae Agallochae (*Chen Xiang*), 4g, Fructus Litchi Sinensis (*Li Zhi Rou*), 7 whole ones

Method of preparation: Place the above 9 ingredients in a large jar, soak in 2 *jin* of alcohol, and seal the lid. Three days later, add 1/4 cup of boiling hot water and also cold water to discharge the fire toxins. Then allow to tincture for another 3 weeks until ready.

Method of administration: Take 1-2 small teacups each morning and evening.

Huang Qi Dang Gui Jiu (Astragalus & *Dang Gui* Wine)

Functions: Supplements the qi and blood, opens the channels and collaterals, dispels wind cold, and transforms phlegm rheum

Mainly treats: Paralysis of the four extremities, swelling and pain all over the body, aversion to cold, phlegm fullness in the chest, aversion to chilled foods and drinks, cold *shan* and abdominal pain, low back pain due to prolonged lying on damp earth, dizziness, tinnitus, or blurred vision when standing up, absentmindedness, poor memory

Ingredients: Radix Astragali Membranacei (*Huang Qi*), 45g, Radix Angelicae Sinensis (*Dang Gui*), 36g, Radix Angelicae Pubescentis (*Du Huo*), 45g, Radix Ledebouriellae Sesloidis (*Fang Feng*), Herba Cum Radice Asari (*Xi Xin*), 45g, Radix Achyranthis Bidentatae (*Niu Xi*), 45g, Rhizoma Ligustici Wallichii (*Chuan Xiong*), 45g, mix-fried Radix Glycyrrhizae (*Zhi Gan Cao*), Radix Praeparatus Aconiti Carmichaeli (*Zhi Fu Zi*), 45g, Fructus Zanthoxyli Bungeani (*Shu Jiao*), 45g, processed Radix Aconiti (*Zhi Chuan Wu*), 30g, Fructus Corni Officinalis (*Shan Zhu Yu*), 30g, dry Radix Puerariae Lobatae (*Gan Ge Gen*), 30g, Radix Gentianae Macrophyllae (*Qin Jiao*), Cortex Cinnamomi (*Guan Gui*), 36g, raw Radix Et Rhizoma Rhei (*Sheng Da Huang*), Rhizoma Atractylodis Macrocephalae (*Bai Zhu*), 15g, dry Rhizoma Zingiberis (*Gan Jiang*), 15g

Method of preparation: Break up the above 18 medicinals into pieces and place in a large jar. Soak in 4 *jin* of alcohol. Seal the opening. Allow to tincture for 5 days in the spring and summer and 7 days in the fall and winter. Then open, discard the dregs, and store for use.

Method of administration: Take 10-30ml each time, 1 time per day until healed. If the person is old and weak, take slightly warm.

Method of modification: If one side of the body is vacuous and weak, add Herba Cistanchis (*Rou Cong Rong*), 30g. If there is poor memory, add Herba Dendrobii (*Shi Hu*), 30g, Rhizoma Acori Graminei (*Shi Chang Pu*), 30g, and Fluoritum (*Zi Shi Ying*), 30g. If there is excessive water below the heart, add Sclerotium Poriae Cocos (*Fu Ling*), 30g, Radix Codonopsis Pilosulae (*Dang Shen*), 30g, and Radix Dioscoreae Oppositae (*Shan Yao*), 45g.

Xi Chun Jiu (Sunny Spring Wine)

Functions: Warms the kidneys and supplements the lungs, moistens the muscles and skin, blackens the hair, restores the color to the cheeks

Mainly treats: Enduring cough in the elderly, lusterless facial color

Ingredients: Fructus Lycii Chinensis (*Gou Qi Zi*), 20g, Arillus Euphoriae Longanae (*Long Yan Rou*), 20g, Fructus Ligustri Lucidi (*Nu Zhen Zi*), 20g, Radix Rehmanniae (*Sheng Di*), 20g, Herba Epimedii (*Yin Yang Huo*), 20g, Semen Phaseoli Munginis (*Lu Dou*), 20g, lard, 100g

Method of preparation: First steam the Ligustrum Lucidum and dry in the sun 9 times. Wash the Rehmannia, Epimedium, and Mung Beans and dry in the sun. Place all the above ingredients in a thin, sturdy silk bag and put this bag in a large jar. Soak this bag in 2kg of alcohol, seal the lid, and allow to tincture for 1 month. Open the lid, remove the bag, and store for use.

Method of administration: Take 15ml each morning and evening.

Bu Yi Qi Guan Jiu (Supplement & Boost Lycium & Cinnamon Wine)

Functions: Supplements the heart and enriches the kidneys, boosts the will and quiets the spirit

Mainly treats: Dizziness, blurred vision, insomnia, excessive dreams

Ingredients: Fructus Lycii Chinensis (*Gou Qi Zi*), 150g, Cortex Cinnamomi (*Rou Gui*), 200g

Method of preparation: Soak the above 2 ingredients in 1kg of white alcohol for 14 days.

Method of administration: Take 20ml each time, 2 times per day.

Wu Xu Jiu (Black Beard Wine)

Functions: Nourishes and supplements the liver and kidneys, blackens the beard, blackens the hair

Mainly treats: Premature greying of the hair. Prolonged use increases the years and boosts longevity.

Ingredients: Radix Polygoni Multiflori (*He Shou Wu*), 500g each of the red and white varieties, Radix Rehmanniae (*Sheng Di*), 120g, Succus Rhizomatis Zingiberis (*Sheng Jiang Zhi, i.e.*, Ginger Juice), 120g, Fructus Zizyphi Jujubae (*Da Zao*), 90g, Semen Juglandis Regiae (*Hu Tao Ren*), 90g, Semen Nelumbinis Nuciferae (*Lian Zi Rou*), 90g, Radix Angelicae Sinensis (*Dang Gui*), 60g, Fructus Lycii Chinensis (*Gou Qi Zi*), 60g, Tuber Ophiopogonis Japonicae (*Mai Men Dong*), 30g

Method of preparation: Soak the above ingredients in 7.5kg of rice wine for 1/2 month. Then remove the dregs and add 90g of Honey.

Method of administration: Take 3 teacups each time at no fixed schedule.

75

5

Wines for Strengthening the Sinews & Bones

Like many of the formulas in the preceding chapter, the formulas in this chapter mostly contain liver blood nourishing and kidney enriching and supplementing ingredients. Therefore, one can say that these formulas form a subcategory of supplementing formulas. As one ages, one's sinews become stiff and bones brittle. In TCM, this is because there is insufficient blood to nourish and moisten the sinews and because there is insufficient essence to fill the marrow. In regard to the sinews and bones, it is said that the liver governs the sinews and the kidneys govern the bones. It is also said that the liver and kidneys share a common source and that the blood and essence share a common source. That common source is the kidney essence in both cases. This reiterates the fact that, in Chinese medicine, it is the kidneys which govern one's physical body as a whole and govern conception, growth, maturation, and aging.

However, unlike the supplementing formulas above which are designed to brighten the eyes, improve the hearing, keep the hair black, and generally retard the aging process, most of the ones in this chapter are designed to emphasize the nourishing of the sinews and the strengthening of the bones. In Chinese medicine, there are disease categories called 40 years shoulder and 50 years wrist. These are muscle/joint pains which are due to vacuity and insufficiency, not to obstruction or blockage. This type of pain is worse after rest and better after movement. This is because movement promotes the flow of qi and blood to the affected area. Once the flow is promoted, the pain subsides. Many of the formulas in this chapter are designed to treat this type of muscle/joint pain.

Other formulas in this chapter do treat *bi* or obstruction pain but due to vacuity. In this case, wind, cold, or dampness may invade the channels and network vessels and affect the sinews and bones because they take advantage of an underlying vacuity of righteous qi. Here there are symptoms of both vacuity and repletion at the same time. Therefore, in these formulas, there are supplementing and nourishing ingredients as well as ingredients to scatter cold, dispel wind, and eliminate dampness.

In addition, one will find in this chapter formulas to treat the sequelae of strokes or what TCM calls wind strike. Although wind strike may be due to internal stirring of wind in turn due to liver fire or hyperactivity of ascendant liver yang, after a stroke the patient is typically vacuous and weak. Therefore, these formulas include ingredients to supplement the qi and nourish the blood, enrich yin and reinforce yang. However, because there may be lingering wind, they may also include ingredients to track down and level wind. And because there may be blood stasis, they may include ingredients that quicken the blood and transform stasis. Thus these formulas tend to be both large and complex in their formulation.

Further, many formulas in this chapter help keep the bones from being brittle due to aging. Osteoporosis is a major concern among older people. Everyone knows some relative or friend whose bones have broken either from bearing one's own weight or due to what otherwise should have been a minor accident. The formulas in this category help to prevent and reverse osteoporosis in the elderly. The fact Chinese kidney-supplementing medicinals which strengthen the sinews and bones are capable of beneficially affecting bone density and strength is corroborated by research done in Japan on post-menopausal women.[1]

---

[1]   *Traditional Sino-Japanese Medicine*, #13, 1992, p. 38-43

Many traditional Chinese formulas for strengthening the sinews and bones contain an ingredient from an endangered species. This refers to Os Tigridis (*Hu Gu*) or Tiger Bone. Although it is said that the Chinese not only use real Tiger Bone but also the bones of other species of cat and even pigs, because the continued use of real Tiger Bone places a high price on this commodity which tempts people to kill these magnificent animals, I have chosen not to include in this book any of the many formulas in this category of Chinese medicinal wines which have Tiger Bone in them. One can still get a good therapeutic effect in terms of strengthening the sinews and bones without using this ingredient.

Because weakness of the sinews and bones is usually a symptom which goes along with aging, those under 60 years of age should use the formulas in this chapter with care. Younger people with various atonic or what TCM refers to as *wei zheng*, paralytic conditions such as MS, lupus, and postpolio sequelae, can often benefit by using the same medicinals as described in these formulas. However, because such patients so frequently also exhibit signs and symptoms of candidiasis, taking these medicinals in a wine or alcohol base is typically counterproductive.

However, for the older person with chronic pain, weakness, or stiffness in their low back, knees, or feet which gets better after movement or as the day goes on or for those who either have osteoporosis or are concerned about osteoporosis, the Chinese medicinal wines in this chapter may be very beneficial. As long as one has the corroborating signs and symptoms of either qi and blood or yin and yang vacuity, they can be used with relative safety and efficacy.

Because many of the formulas in this chapter contain yang supplements and warming ingredients, patients with any hot signs or symptoms, whether that be due to internal heat, vacuity heat, or stirring of life gate fire should get a diagnosis and prescription from a qualified professional TCM practitioner before self-medicating with any of the wines in this chapter.

Huang Qi Shi Hu Jiu (Astragalus & Dendrobium Wine)

Functions: Supports the righteous and eliminates wind

Mainly treats: Righteous vacuity and wind invasion, low back and lower leg *bi* pain, numbness and *bi* of the cheeks and face

Ingredients: Herba Dendrobii (*Shi Hu*), 120g, Radix Astragali Membranacei (*Huang Qi*), 45g, Radix Codonopsis Pilosulae (*Dang Shen*), 45g, Radix Ledebouriellae Sesloidis (*Fang Feng*), 45g, Radix Salviae Miltiorrhizae (*Dan Shen*), 60g, Fructus Corni Officinalis (*Shan Zhu Yu*), 60g, Cortex Eucommiae Ulmoidis (*Du Zhong*), 60g, Radix Achyranthis Bidentatae (*Niu Xi*), 60g, Herba Cum Radice Asari (*Xi Xin*), 30g, Tuber Asparagi Cochinensis (*Tian Men Dong*), 70g, raw Rhizoma Zingiberis (*Sheng Jiang*), 90g, Semen Coicis Lachryma-jobi (*Yi Yi Ren*), 150g, Fructus Lycii Chinensis (*Gou Qi Zi*), 150g, Fructus Schizandrae Chinensis (*Wu Wei Zi*), 60g, Sclerotium Poriae Cocos (*Fu Ling*), 60g, Radix Dioscoreae Oppositae (*Shan Yao*), 60g, Rhizoma Dioscoreae Hypoglaucae (*Bi Xie*), 60g

Method of preparation: Grind the above 17 medicinals into powder and place in a large jar. Soak in 6 *jin* of yellow wine (*i.e.*, rice wine) for 5 days and then open. Remove the dregs and store for use.

Method of administration: Take 2-3 teacups per day. In order to get the strength of this wine, it is important to take it continuously without stopping for a period of time.

80

Dan Shen Shi Hu Jiu (Salvia & Dendrobium Wine)

Functions: Supplements vacuity and dispels evils, quickens the blood and stops pain

Mainly treats: Foot qi *bi* and weakness, aching and pain of the sinews and bones

Ingredients: Herba Dendrobii (*Shi Hu*), 60g, Radix Salviae Miltior-rhizae (*Dan Shen*), 30g, Rhizoma Ligustici Wallichii (*Chuan Xiong*), 30g, Cortex Eucommiae Ulmoidis (*Du Zhong*), 30g, Radix Ledebour-iellae Sesloidis (*Fang Feng*), 30g, Rhizoma Atractylodis Macroce-phalae (*Bai Zhu*), 30g, Radix Codonopsis Pilosulae (*Dang Shen*), 30g, Cortex Cinnamomi (*Rou Gui*), 30g, Fructus Schizandrae Chinensis (*Wu Wei Zi*), 30g, Sclerotium Poriae Cocos (*Fu Ling*), 30g, Pericar-pium Citri Reticulatae (*Chen Pi*), 30g, Radix Astragali Membranacei (*Huang Qi*), 30g, dry Rhizoma Zingiberis (*Gan Jiang*), 45g, mix-fried Radix Glycyrrhizae (*Zhi Gan Cao*), 15g, Radix Dioscoreae Oppositae (*Shan Yao*), 30g, Radix Achyranthis Bidentatae (*Niu Xi*), 45g, Radix Angelicae Sinensis (*Dang Gui*), 30g

Method of preparation: Grind the above 17 ingredients into a fine powder and place in a large jar. Soak in 4 *jin* of clear alcohol and seal the lid. Open after 7 days and remove the dregs. Store for use.

Method of administration: Take 1-2 teacups warm before meals 2 times per day.

Niu Xi Shi Hu Jiu (Achyranthes & Dendrobium Wine)

Functions: Dispels wind and overcomes dampness, supplements the kidneys and strengthens the low back, strengthens the bones

Mainly treats: Wind, cold, damp qi *bi* obstructing the low back and lower legs, feebleness, weakness, and lack of strength, numbness and insensitivity

Ingredients: Herba Dendrobii (*Shi Hu*), 85g, Radix Achyranthis Bidentatae (*Niu Xi*), 15g, Cortex Eucommiae Ulmoidis (*Du Zhong*), 120g, Radix Salviae Miltiorrhizae (*Dan Shen*), 90g, prepared Radix Rehmanniae (*Shu Di*), 150g, Cortex Cinnamomi (*Rou Gui*), 60g

Method of preparation: Grind the above six medicinals into a fine powder and place in a large jar. Soak in 4 *jin* of alcohol and seal the lid. Then put the jar in a pan of water and bring to a boil 100 times. Open the lid, remove the dregs, and store for use.

Method of administration: Take 1-2 teacups each time warm at no fixed intervals. Usually it will make one just slightly tipsy.

Fu Ling Ju Hua Jiu (Poria & Chrysanthemum Wine)

Functions: Dispels wind qi, disinhibits the joints, strengthens the sinews and bones, warms the liver and kidneys

Mainly treats: Soreness and pain of the joints of the bones, difficulty moving, pain on movement especially of the shoulders and upper back, paralysis of one half of the body, aphasia due to wind stroke

Ingredients: Sclerotium Poriae Cocos (*Fu Ling*), 40g, Flos Chrysanthemi Morifolii (*Gan Ju Hua*), Fructus Corni Officinalis (*Shan Zhu Yu*), 15g, Semen Cuscutae (*Tu Si Zi*), 22g, Herba Cistanchis (*Rou Cong Rong*), 15g, Radix Trichosanthis Kirlowii (*Tian Hua Fen*), 15g, Radix Ledebouriellae Sesloidis (*Fang Feng*), 15g, prepared Radix Rehmanniae (*Shu Di*), 15g, Cortex Radicis Moutan (*Dan Pi*), 15g, Radix Panacis Ginseng (*Ren Shen*), 10g, Rhizoma Atractylodis

Macrocephalae (*Bai Zhu*), 10g, Concha Ostreae (*Mu Li*), 15g, Semen Cnidii Monnieri (*She Chuang Zi*), 10g, Radix Astragali Membranacei (*Huang Qi*), 15g, Radix Asteris Tatarici (*Zi Wan*), 10g, Rhizoma Acori Graminei (*Shi Chang Pu*), 15g, Herba Dendrobii (*Shi Hu*), 10g, Semen Biotae Orientalis (*Bai Zi Ren*), 120g, Cortex Eucommiae Ulmoidis (*Du Zhong*), 15g, Radix Polygalae Tenuifoliae (*Yuan Zhi*), 15g, Radix Praeparatus Aconiti Carmichaeli (*Zhi Fu Zi*), 15g, dry Rhizoma Zingiberis (*Gan Jiang*), 15g, Radix Rubrus Paeoniae Lactiflorae (*Chi Shao*), 15g, Radix Achyranthis Bidentatae (*Niu Xi*), 15g, Rhizoma Dioscoreae Hypoglaucae (*Bi Xie*), 15g, Rhizoma Cibotii Barometsis (*Gou Ji*), 15g, Fructus Xanthii (*Cang Er Zi*), 15g, stir-fried Fructus Arctii Lappae (*Niu Bang Zi*), 10g, Radix Platycodi Grandiflori (*Jie Geng*), 10g, Radix Et Rhizoma Notopterygii (*Qiang Huo*), Fructus Lycii Chinensis (*Gou Qi Zi*), 10g, Radix Dipsaci (*Xu Duan*), 15g, Radix Arctii Lappae (*Niu Bang Gen, i.e.,* Burdock Root), 15g, Bombyx Batryticatus (*Can Sha*), 22g

Method of preparation: Grind the above 35 ingredients into a fine powder and place in a large jar. Soak in 4 *jin* of alcohol and seal the lid. Allow to tincture for 15 days. Then open the lid, remove the dregs, and store for use.

Method of administration: Take 1 small teacup warm each morning, noon, and night.

Niu Xi Dan Shen Jiu (Achyranthes & Salvia Wine)

Functions: Scatters cold and dispels wind, supplements fire and rescues yang, soothes the sinews and quickens the blood, warms the middle and stops pain

Mainly treats: Prolonged summer low back and lower leg *bi* and weakness, aching and pain of the sinews and bones which cannot be

83

bent, numbness and insensitivity of the skin, swelling and pain of the joints of the fingers and toes

Ingredients: Radix Achyranthis Bidentatae (*Niu Xi*), 25g, Radix Salviae Miltiorrhizae (*Dan Shen*), 25g, Semen Coicis Lachryma-jobi (*Yi Yi Ren*), 25g, raw Radix Rehmanniae (*Sheng Di*), 25g, Cortex Radicis Acanthopanacis (*Wu Jia Pi*), 18g, Rhizoma Atractylodis Macrocephalae (*Bai Zhu*), 18g, Radix Praeparatus Aconiti Carmichaeli (*Fu Zi*), 12g, Rhizoma Dioscoreae Hypoglaucae (*Bi Xie*), 12g, Sclerotium Rubrum Poriae Cocos (*Chi Fu Ling*), 12g, Radix Ledebouriellae Sesloidis (*Fang Feng*), 12g, Radix Angelicae Pubescentis (*Du Huo*), 20g, Herba Dendrobii (*Shi Hu*), 20g, Caulis Piperis Kadsurae (*Hai Feng Teng*), 10g, Cortex Cinnamomi (*Rou Gui*), 10g, Radix Panacis Ginseng (*Ren Shen*), 10g, Rhizoma Ligustici Wallichii (*Chuan Xiong*), 10g, Folium Photiniae Serrulatae (*Shi Nan Ye*), 10g, Herba Cum Radice Asari (*Xi Xin*), 6g, Rhizoma Cimicifugae (*Sheng Ma*), 6g, Magnetitum (*Ci Shi*), 50g, raw Rhizoma Zingiberis (*Sheng Jiang*), 15g

Method of administration: Grind the above 21 medicinals into a fine powder and place in a large jar. Soak in 3 *jin* of clear alcohol and seal the lid. After 7 days, open the lid, remove the dregs, and store for use.

Method of administration: Take 1 teacup on an empty stomach 5 times per day. For those who do not like to drink alcohol or are not used to drinking alcohol, they may drink this wine fewer times and still get some result.

Niu Xi Ren Shen Jiu (Achyranthes & Ginseng Wine)

Functions: Supplements fire and rescues yang, warms the center and stops pain, strengthens the sinews and bones

84

Mainly treats: Low back and lower leg aching and pain, chilly vacuity of the lower origin, impotence and spermatorrhea, loose stools and abdominal pain, qi vacuity and lack of strength

Ingredients: Radix Achyranthis Bidentatae (*Niu Xi*), 20g, Fructus Corni Officinalis (*Shan Zhu Yu*), 20g, Rhizoma Ligustici Wallichii (*Chuan Xiong*), 20g, Radix Praeparatus Aconiti Carmichaeli (*Zhi Fu Zi*), 20g, Radix Morindae Officinalis (*Ba Ji Tian*), 20g, Fructus Schizandrae Chinensis (*Wu Wei Zi*), 20g, Radix Astragali Membranacei (*Huang Qi*), 20g, Radix Panacis Ginseng (*Ren Shen*), 20g, Cortex Radicis Acanthopanacis (*Wu Jia Pi*), 25g, Herba Cistanchis (*Rou Cong Rong*), 25g, raw Rhizoma Zingiberis (*Sheng Jiang*), 25g, Radix Ledebouriellae Sesloidis (*Fang Feng*), 25g, Cortex Cinnamomi (*Rou Gui*), 15g, Caulis Piperis Kadsurae (*Hai Feng Teng*), 10g, raw Radix Rehmanniae (*Sheng Di*), 15g, Fructus Zanthoxyli Bungeani (*Shu Jiao*), 15g, Magnetitum (*Ci Shi*), 20g

Method of preparation: Grind the above 17 ingredients into a fine powder and place in a large jar. Soak in 3 *jin* of limeless alcohol. Seal the lid and allow to tincture for 3 days in the spring and summer and 7 days in the fall and winter. Open, remove the dregs, and store for use.

Method of administration: Take 15-20ml slightly warm each day at no fixed times.

Niu Xi Rou Gui Jiu (Achyranthes & Cinnamon Wine)

Functions: Supplements the kidneys and strengthens yang, dispels wind and eliminates dampness

Mainly treats: Low back and knee soreness and weakness, impotence and spermatorrhea, loose stools, vacuity swelling of the lower legs and

85

feet, aching and pain of the joints, lack of warmth in the four limbs, chilly pain in the abdominal region

Ingredients: Radix Achyranthis Bidentatae (*Niu Xi*), 30g, Radix Gentianae Macrophyllae (*Qin Jiao*), 30g, Rhizoma Ligustici Wallichii (*Chuan Xiong*), 30g, Radix Ledebouriellae Sesloidis (*Fang Feng*), 30g, Cortex Cinnamomi (*Rou Gui*), 30g, Radix Angelicae Pubescentis (*Du Huo*), 30g, Radix Salviae Miltiorrhizae (*Dan Shen*), 30g, Sclerotium Poriae Cocos (*Fu Ling*), 30g, Cortex Eucommiae Ulmoidis (*Du Zhong*), 25g, Radix Praeparatus Aconiti Carmichaeli (*Zhi Fu Zi*), 25g, Herba Dendrobii (*Shi Hu*), 25g, dry Rhizoma Zingiberis (*Gan Jiang*), 25g, Tuber Ophiopogonis Japonicae (*Mai Men Dong*), 25g, Cortex Radicis Lycii (*Di Gu Pi*), 25g, Cortex Radicis Acanthopanacis (*Wu Jia Pi*), 40g, Semen Coicis Lachryma-jobi (*Yi Yi Ren*), 15g, Semen Cannabis Sativae (*Huo Ma Ren*), 10g

Method of preparation: Grind the above 17 ingredients into a fine powder and place in a large jar. Soak in 3 *jin* of clear alcohol and seal the lid. Allow to tincture for 3 days in the spring and summer and for 7 days in the fall and winter. Open, remove the dregs, and decant.

Method of administration: Take 15ml each time warm on an empty stomach 3 times per day.

Niu Xi Yu Mi Jiu (Achyranthes Jade Rice Wine)

Functions: Dispels wind, scatters cold, and eliminates dampness, boosts the liver and kidneys, rescues yang and supplements fire, soothes the sinews and vessels, disinhibits the joints

Mainly treats: Numbness and insensitivity of the fingers of the hand, chilly pain of the low back and knees, sinew and vessel spasms, inhibited joints of the limbs, loose stools, essence spirit debility and decline

Ingredients: Radix Achyranthis Bidentatae (*Niu Xi*), 30g, Semen Coicis Lachryma-jobi (*Yi Yi Ren*), 30g, Semen Zizyphi Spinosae (*Suan Zao Ren*), 30g, Radix Rubrus Paeoniae Lactiflorae (*Chi Shao*), 30g, Radix Praeparatus Aconiti Carmichaeli (*Zhi Fu Zi*), 30g, blast-fried Rhizoma Zingiberis (*Pao Jiang*), 30g, Herba Dendrobii (*Shi Hu*), 30g, Semen Biotae Orientalis (*Bai Zi Ren*), 30g, mix-fried Radix Glycyrrhizae (*Zhi Gan Cao*), 20g

Method of preparation: Grind the above 9 ingredients into a fine powder and place in a large jar. Soak in 3 *jin* of alcohol and seal the lid. After 7 days, open, remove the dregs, and store for use.

Method of administration: Take 15-20ml warm at no fixed times.

Niu Xi Fu Zi Jiu (Achyranthes & Aconite Wine)

Functions: Scatters cold and dispels wind, supplements fire and rescues yang, soothes the sinews and quickens the blood, warms the center and stops pain

Mainly treats: Numbness and insensitivity of the fingers of the hands, low back and knee soreness and pain, difficulty walking, weak feet, spasms and cramps, lack of warmth of the four limbs, possible impotence, loose stools, soreness and pain of the muscles and flesh

Ingredients: Radix Achyranthis Bidentatae (*Niu Xi*), 15g, Radix Gentianae Macrophyllae (*Qin Jiao*), 15g, Tuber Asparagi Cochinensis (*Tian Men Dong*), 15g, Semen Coicis Lachryma-jobi (*Yi Yi Ren*), 10g, Radix Angelicae Pubescentis (*Du Huo*), mix-fried Herba Cum Radice Asari (*Zhi Xi Xin*), 10g, Radix Praeparatus Aconiti Carmichaeli (*Zhi*

Fu Zi), 10g, Radix Morindae Officinalis (*Ba Ji Tian*), 10g, Cortex Radicis Acanthopanacis (*Wu Jia Pi*), 15g, Cortex Cinnamomi (*Rou Gui*), 10g, Cortex Eucommiae Ulmoidis (*Du Zhong*), 15g, Folium Photiniae Serrulatae (*Shi Nan Ye*), 10g

Method of preparation: Grind the above 12 medicinals into a fine powder and place in a large jar. Soak in 2 *jin* of clear alcohol for 10 days in winter, 7 days in spring, 5 days in fall, and 3 days in summer. After tincturing, remove the dregs and decant.

Method of administration: Take 15ml each time, 3 times per day, morning, noon, and night.

Cong Zi Jiu (Semen Allii Fistulosi Wine)

Functions: Supplements the kidney qi, strengthens the low back and knees, eliminates wind and dispels cold

Mainly treats: Kidney vacuity low back and knee aching and pain possibly reaching to the lower legs and feet, spasms of the lower and upper back when bending backward, inhibition of bending forward

Ingredients: Semen Allii Fistulosi (*Cong Zi*), 20g, Cortex Eucommiae Ulmoidis (*Du Zhong*), Radix Achyranthis Bidentatae (*Niu Xi*), 20g, Herba Epimedii (*Xian Ling Pi*), 15g, Zaocys Dhumnades (*Wu She*), 30g, Herba Dendrobii (*Shi Hu*), 20g, Radix Praeparatus Aconiti Carmichaeli (*Zhi Fu Zi*), 20g, Radix Ledebouriellae Sesloidis (*Fang Feng*), 20g, Cortex Cinnamomi (*Rou Gui*), 20g, Rhizoma Ligustici Wallichii (*Chuan Xiong*), 15g, Fructus Zanthoxyli Bungeani (*Chuan Jiao*), 15g, Rhizoma Atractylodis Macrocephalae (*Bai Zhu*), 20g, Cortex Radicis Acanthopanacis (*Wu Jia Pi*), 20g, stir-fried Semen Zizyphi Spinosae (*Chao Zao Ren*), 20g

Method of preparation: Pestle the above 14 ingredients into a coarse powder and place in a large jar. Soak in 3 *jin* of alcohol and seal the lid. After 7 days, open, remove the dregs, and store for use.

Method of administration: Take 1 small teacup warm before each meal.

Huang Qi Du Zhong Jiu (Astragalus & Eucommia Wine)

Functions: Warms and supplements kidney yang, strengthens the low back and knees

Mainly treats: Kidney yang vacuity detriment, timid qi and fatigued spirit, chilly pain in the low back and knees, impotence and spermatorrhea

Ingredients: Radix Astragali Membranacei (*Huang Qi*), 30g, Rhizoma Dioscoreae Hypoglaucae (*Bi Xie*), 45g, Radix Ledebouriellae Sesloidis (*Fang Feng*), 45g, Radix Achyranthis Bidentatae (*Niu Xi*), 60g, Cortex Cinnamomi (*Rou Gui*), 30g, Herba Dendrobii (*Shi Hu*), 60g, Cortex Eucommiae Ulmoidis (*Du Zhong*), 45g, Herba Cistanchis (*Rou Cong Rong*), 60g, Radix Praeparatus Aconiti Carmichaeli (*Zhi Fu Zi*), 30g, Fructus Corni Officinalis (*Shan Zhu Yu*), 30g, Folium Photiniae Serrulatae (*Shi Non Ye*), 30g, Sclerotium Poriae Cocos (*Fu Ling*), 30g

Method of preparation: Grind the above 12 ingredients into a fine powder and place in a large jar. Soak in 3.5 *jin* of alcohol for 3 days. Remove the dregs and decant.

Method of administration: Take 1-2 teacups warm before each meal.

Ba Wei Huang Qi Jiu (Eight Flavors Astragalus Wine)

Functions: Supplements the qi and boosts vacuity, strengthens the low back and knees, harmonizes the blood vessels

Mainly treats: Yang qi vacuity weakness, chilly counterflow of the hands and feet, aching and pain of the low back and knees

Ingredients: Radix Astragali Membranacei (*Huang Qi*), 60g, Rhizoma Dioscoreae Hypoglaucae (*Bi Xie*), 45g, Radix Ledebouriellae Sesloidis (*Fang Feng*), 45g, Rhizoma Ligustici Wallichii (*Chuan Xiong*), 45g, Radix Achyranthis Bidentatae (*Niu Xi*), 45g, Radix Angelicae Pubescentis (*Du Huo*), 30g, Fructus Corni Officinalis (*Shan Zhu Yu*), 30g, Fructus Schizandrae Chinensis (*Wu Wei Zi*), 60g

Method of preparation: Grind the above 8 ingredients into a fine powder and place in a large jar. Soak in 3 *jin* of alcohol. Allow to tincture for 5 days in the fall and winter and for 3 days in the spring and summer. Open the lid, remove the dregs, and store for use.

Method of administration: Take 1-2 teacups warm on an empty stomach each day.

Liang Pi Du Huo Jiu (Two Peels Angelica Pubescens Wine)

Functions: Warms the kidneys and dispels winds, strengthens the low back and the bones

Mainly treats: Feebleness, weakness, aching, and pain of the feet and knees, numbness of the four limbs, inhibition of the joints, inability to flex and bend

90

Ingredients: Cortex Erythrinae Variegatae (*Hai Tong Pi*), 30g, Cortex Radicis Acanthopanacis (*Wu Jia Pi*), 30g, Radix Angelicae Pubescentis (*Du Huo*), 30g, Radix Praeparatus Aconiti Carmichaeli (*Zhi Fu Zi*), 10g, Herba Dendrobii (*Shi Hu*), 30g, Cortex Cinnamomi (*Rou Gui*), 30g, Radix Ledebouriellae Sesloidis (*Fang Feng*), 30g, Radix Angelicae Sinensis (*Dang Gui*), 30g, Cortex Eucommiae Ulmoidis (*Du Zhong*), 30g, Herba Epimedii (*Xian Ling Pi*), 30g, Rhizoma Dioscoreae Hypoglaucae (*Bi Xie*), 30g, Radix Achyranthis Bidentatae (*Niu Xi*), 30g, Semen Coicis Lachryma-jobi (*Yi Yi Ren*), 30g, raw Radix Rehmanniae (*Sheng Di*), 30g

Method of preparation: Grind the above 14 medicinals into a fine powder and place in a large jar. Soak in 3 *jin* of white alcohol for 7 days in the spring and summer and for 14 days in the fall and winter. Remove the dregs and store for use.

Method of administration: Take 1-2 teacups warm on an empty stomach. It is normal to feel a little tipsy. However, one should not get drunk. One should not use more than one refill of this formula.

Niu Xi Bai Zhu Jiu (Achyranthes & Atractylodes Wine)

Functions: Reinforces yang and scatters cold, dispels wind and disinhibits dampness, strengthens the sinews and bones, harmonizes the blood vessels

Mainly treats: Soreness and pain of the low back and knees, difficulty walking, weak feet, inhibited joints, dizziness and vertigo, lack of warmth in the four limbs

Ingredients: Radix Achyranthis Bidentatae (*Niu Xi*), 15g, Radix Praeparatus Aconiti Carmichaeli (*Zhi Fu Zi*), 15g, Radix Salviae Miltiorrhizae (*Dan Shen*), 15g, Fructus Corni Officinalis (*Shan Zhu*

Yu), 15g, Caulis Et Folium Sambucudis Javanicae (*Liu Ying*), 15g, Cortex Eucommiae Ulmoidis (*Du Zhong*), 15g, Herba Dendrobii (*Shi Hu*), 15g, Radix Ledebouriellae Sesloidis (*Fang Feng*), 12g, Fructus Zanthoxyli Bungeani (*Shu Jiao*), 12g, Herba Cum Radice Asari (*Xi Xin*), 12g, Radix Angelicae Pubescentis (*Du Huo*), 12g, Radix Gentianae Macrophyllae (*Qin Jiao*), 12g, Cortex Cinnamomi (*Rou Gui*),12g, Semen Coicis Lachryma-jobi (*Yi Yi Ren*), 12g, Rhizoma Ligustici Wallichii (*Chuan Xiong*), 12g, Radix Angelicae Sinensis (*Dang Gui*), 20g, Rhizoma Atractylodis Macrocephalae (*Bai Zhu*), 20g, Caulis et Folium Skimmiae Reevesianae (*Yin Yu*), 15g, Cortex Radicis Acanthopanacis (*Wu Jia Pi*), 20g, blast-fried Rhizoma Zingiberis (*Pao Jiang*), 10g

Method of preparation: Grind the above 20 medicinals into a fine powder and place in a large jar. Soak in 3 *jin* of clear alcohol and seal the lid. Allow to tincture for 7 days in the winter and for 3 days in the summer. Then open the lid, remove the dregs, and decant.

Method of administration: Begin by take 15ml each time and increase the amount as long as one feels normal. If one feels dizzy, then reduce the amount.

Note: This formula may be taken for a long time.

Xian Mao Jia Pi Jiu (Curculigo & Acanthopanax Wine)

Functions: Supplements the liver and boosts the kidneys, reinforces yang and strengthens the body, scatters cold and eliminates *bi*

Mainly treats: Spasms and cramps in the sinews and vessels of the low back and knees, numbness of the muscles and skin, inhibited joints, impotence, cold, frigid uterus infertility

Ingredients: Rhizoma Curculiginis Orchoidis (*Xian Mao*), 90g, Herba Epimedii (*Yin Yang Huo*), 120g, Cortex Radicis Acanthopanacis (*Wu Jia Pi*), 90g

Method of preparation: Grind the above medicinals into a fine powder and place in a small jug of mellow alcohol (*i.e.* brandy or sherry). Seal the lid and soak for 7 days. Then open and decant.

Method of administration: Take 1-2 teacups each morning and evening.

Xian Mao Jiu (Curculigo Wine)

Functions: Warms the kidneys and reinforces yang, dispels cold and eliminates dampness

Mainly treats: Impotence and spermatorrhea, chilly pain of the low back and knees, cold sperm in men, frigid uterus infertility in women, urinary incontinence in the elderly, terminal dribbling

Ingredients: Rhizoma Curculiginis Orchoidis (*Xian Mao*), 120g

Method of preparation: Steam the Curculigo 9 times and dry in the sun 9 times alternately. Then place in a large jar and soak in 1 *jin* of alcohol. Seal the lid. After 7 days, open, remove the dregs, and store for use.

Method of administration: Take 15-20ml on an empty stomach each morning and evening.

Contraindications: This formula is not appropriate if there is ministerial fire effulgence and exuberance.

Gou Ji Jiu (Cibotium Wine)

Functions: Quickens the blood and opens the network vessels, supplements the liver and boosts the kidneys, dispels wind and disinhibits dampness, strengthens the sinews and bones

Mainly treats: Stubborn pain of the lower and upper back, inhibited bending and flexing, feeble feet and lack of strength, urinary incontinence, excessive abnormal vaginal discharge, numbness, aching and pain in the body and limbs, inhibited joints

Ingredients: Rhizoma Cibotii Barometsis (*Gou Ji*), 18g, Radix Salviae Miltiorrhizae (*Dan Shen*), 18g, Radix Astragali Membranacei (*Huang Qi*), 18g, Rhizoma Dioscoreae Hypoglaucae (*Bi Xie*), 18g, Radix Achyranthis Bidentatae (*Niu Xi*), 18g, Rhizoma Ligustici Wallichii (*Chuan Xiong*), 18g, Radix Angelicae Pubescentis (*Du Huo*), 18g, Radix Praeparatus Aconiti Carmichaeli (*Zhi Fu Zi*), 12g

Method of preparation: Grind the above 8 ingredients into a fine powder and place in a large jar. Soak in 2 *jin* of alcohol and seal the lid. Place this in a pot of water and bring to a rolling boil. Remove and allow to cool. Then open and decant.

Method of administration: Take whatever amount one wishes at no fixed schedule.

Ling Pi Di Huang Jiu (Epimedium & Rehmannia Wine)

Functions: Supplements the kidneys and reinforces yang, dispels wind and dampness, strengthens the sinews and bones

Mainly treats: Kidney vacuity impotence, frigid uterus infertility, lack of strength of the low back and knees, soreness and pain of the sinews and bones

Ingredients: Herba Epimedii (*Xian Ling Pi*), 250g, prepared Radix Rehmanniae (*Shu Di*), 150g

Method of preparation: Grind the above two ingredients into a fine powder and place in a large jar. Soak in 2.5 *jin* of mellow wine and seal the lid. Allow to tincture for 3 days in the spring and summer and for 5 days in the fall and winter. Then open and decant.

Method of administration: Each day take whatever amount one wants warm. It is normal to feel the wine qi slightly (*i.e.*, to feel just a bit tipsy or high), but one should not get drunk.

Xian Ling Pi Jiu (Epimedium Wine)

Functions: Supplements the kidneys and reinforces yang, dispels wind and eliminates dampness, strengthens the sinews and bones

Mainly treats: Feebleness, weakness, and lack of strength of the low back and lower legs, impotence and premature ejaculation

Ingredients: Herba Epimedii (*Xian Ling Pi*), 250g

Method of preparation: Slice the Epimedium into pieces and place in a large jar. Soak in 2 *jin* of white alcohol and seal the lid. After 3 days, open and decant.

Method of administration: Take 1 teacup 3 times per day on an empty stomach.

Fu Zi Du Zhong Jiu (Aconite & Eucommia Wine)

Functions: Warms the yang and opens the interior, scatters cold and dispels dampness, strengthens the low back and boosts the kidneys

Mainly treats: Physical vacuity and weakness after a cold or flu, aching and pain of the low back and knees, difficulty walking and moving about

Ingredients: Cortex Eucommiae Ulmoidis (*Du Zhong*), 50g, Herba Epimedii (*Xian Ling Pi*), 15g, Radix Angelicae Pubescentis (*Du Huo*), 25g, Radix Achyranthis Bidentatae (*Niu Xi*), 25g, Radix Praeparatus Aconiti Carmichaeli (*Zhi Fu Zi*), 30g

Method of preparation: Grind the above ingredients into a fine powder and soak in 2 *jin* of alcohol. After 7 days, open the lid and decant.

Method of administration: Take 10-20ml each time 3 times per day.

Chuan Wu Du Zhong Jiu (*Chuan Wu* Aconite & Eucommia Wine)

Functions: Supplements the kidneys and reinforces yang, strengthens the low back and stops pain

Mainly treats: Kidney vacuity low back pain, wind cold low back pain, low back pain due to prolonged lying on damp earth, low back pain due to injury from lifting a heavy object

Ingredients: Cortex Eucommiae Ulmoidis (*Du Zhong*), 40g, Radix Et Rhizoma Notopterygii (*Qiang Huo*), 40g, blast-fried Rhizoma

Zingiberis (*Pao Jiang*), 20g, Radix Praeparatus Aconiti Carmichaeli (*Zhi Fu Zi*), 40g, Rhizoma Dioscoreae Hypoglaucae (*Bi Xie*), 40g, Cortex Radicis Lycii (*Di Gu Pi*), 30g, Fructus Zanthoxyli Bungeani (*Chuan Jiao*), 15g, Cortex Cinnamomi (*Rou Gui*), 30g, Rhizoma Ligustici Wallichii (*Chuan Xiong*), 30g, Cortex Radicis Acanthopanacis (*Wu Jia Pi*), 40g, Radix Dipsaci (*Xu Duan*), 40g, mix-fried Radix Glycyrrhizae (*Zhi Gan Cao*), 20g, Radix Trichosanthis Kirlowii (*Tian Hua Fen*), 20g, Radix Gentianae Macrophyllae (*Qin Jiao*), 30g, Herba Dendrobii (*Shi Hu*), 30g, processed Radix Aconiti (*Zhi Wu Tou*), 30g, Radix Platycodi Grandiflori (*Jie Geng*), 30g, Herba Cum Radice Asari (*Xi Xin*), 25g, Radix Ledebouriellae Sesloidis (*Fang Feng*), 40g

Method of preparation: Grind the above 19 medicinals into a fine powder and place in a large jar. Soak in 4 *jin* of alcohol and seal the lid. After 5 days, open and decant.

Method of administration: Take 1 medium teacup warm before meals.

Bi Xie Du Zhong Jiu (Dioscorea Hypoglauca & Eucommia Wine)

Functions: Warms and supplements the liver and kidneys, dispels wind and eliminates dampness

Mainly treats: Kidney viscus vacuity chill, possible invasion of cold dampness, chilly *bi* of the low back and lower legs, aching and pain in the bones of the leg

Ingredients: Cortex Eucommiae Ulmoidis (*Du Zhong*), 30g, blast-fried Rhizoma Zingiberis (*Pao Jiang*), 30g, Rhizoma Dioscoreae Hypoglaucae (*Bi Xie*), 30g, Radix Et Rhizoma Notopterygii (*Qiang Huo*), 30g, Radix Praeparatus Aconiti Carmichaeli (*Zhi Fu Zi*), 30g,

Fructus Zanthoxyli Bungeani (*Shu Jiao*), 30g, Cortex Cinnamomi (*Rou Gui*), 30g, Rhizoma Ligustici Wallichii (*Chuan Xiong*), 30g, Radix Ledebouriellae Sesloidis (*Fang Feng*), 30g, Radix Gentianae Macrophyllae (*Qin Jiao*), 30g, mix-fried Radix Glycyrrhizae (*Zhi Gan Cao*), 30g, Herba Cum Radice Asari (*Xi Xin*), 15g, Cortex Radicis Acanthopanacis (*Wu Jia Pi*), 15g, Herba Dendrobii (*Shi Hu*), 15g, Radix Dipsaci (*Xu Duan*), 15g, Cortex Radicis Lycii (*Di Gu Pi*), 15g, Radix Platycodi Grandiflori (*Jie Geng*), 35g

Method of preparation: Grind the above 17 medicinals into a fine powder and place in a large jar. Soak in 3 *jin* of alcohol and seal the lid. Then put this jar into a pot of water and bring to a rolling boil 2 times. Remove, allow to cool, and store for use.

Method of administration: Take 1 teacup warm each time at no fixed schedule. It is normal to feel a little wine qi.

Dan Shen Du Zhong Jiu (Salvia & Eucommia Wine)

Functions: Quickens the blood and opens the network vessels, boosts the liver and supplements the kidneys

Mainly treats: Soreness and pain of the low back and lower legs

Ingredients: Cortex Eucommiae Ulmoidis (*Du Zhong*), 30g, Radix Salviae Miltiorrhizae (*Dan Shen*), 30g, Rhizoma Ligustici Wallichii (*Chuan Xiong*), 20g

Method of preparation: Grind the above 3 ingredients into a fine powder and place in a large jar. Soak in 1.5 *jin* of red rice wine. After 5 nights, remove the dregs and store for use.

Method of administration: Take any amount one wishes at no fixed schedule.

Shu Di Du Zhong Jiu (Prepared Rehmannia & Eucommia Wine)

Functions: Supplements the liver and boosts the kidneys, strengthens the low back and reinforces the entire body

Mainly treats: Aching and pain in the low back region, inability to bend or flex

Ingredients: Mix-fried Cortex Eucommiae Ulmoidis (*Zhi Du Zhong*), 30g, blast-fried Rhizoma Zingiberis (*Pao Jiang*), 30g, prepared Radix Rehmanniae (*Shu Di*), 30g, Rhizoma Dioscoreae Hypoglaucae (*Bi Xie*), 30g, Radix Et Rhizoma Notopterygii (*Qiang Huo*), 30g, Radix Praeparatus Aconiti Carmichaeli (*Zhi Fu Zi*), 30g, Fructus Zanthoxyli Bungeani (*Shu Jiao*), 30g, Cortex Cinnamomi (*Rou Gui*), 30g, Rhizoma Ligustici Wallichii (*Chuan Xiong*), 30g, Radix Aconiti (*Wu Tou*), 30g, Radix Gentianae Macrophyllae (*Qin Jiao*), 30g, Herba Cum Radice Asari (*Xi Xin*), 30g, Cortex Radicis Acanthopanacis (*Wu Jia Pi*), 50g, Herba Dendrobii (*Shi Hu*), 50g, Radix Dipsaci (*Xu Duan*), 30g, Radix Trichosanthis Kirlowii (*Tian Hua Fen*), 25g, Cortex Radicis Lycii (*Di Gu Pi*), 25g, Radix Platycodi Grandiflori (*Jie Geng*), 25g, mix-fried Radix Glycyrrhizae (*Zhi Gan Cao*), 25g, Radix Ledebouriellae Sesloidis (*Fang Feng*), 25g

Method of preparation: Grind the above 20 ingredients into a fine powder and place in a large jar. Soak in 4 *jin* of alcohol. After 4 nights, open the lid, remove the dregs, and store for use.

Method of administration: Take 1 small teacup at no fixed schedule. It is normal to feel a little wine qi.

99

Niu Xi Jia Pi Jiu (Achyranthes & Acanthopanax Wine)

Functions: Strengthens the sinews and bones, supplements the kidneys and boosts yang

Mainly treats: Kidney yang vacuity detriment, wind dampness low back pain, atony and weakness of the legs, aching and pain of the joints and bones

Ingredients: Cortex Radicis Acanthopanacis (*Wu Jia Pi*), 30g, Fructus Citri Seu Ponciri (*Zhi Qiao*), 30g, Radix Angelicae Pubescentis (*Du Huo*), 30g, processed Radix Aconiti (*Zhi Cao Wu*), 30g, blast-fried Rhizoma Zingiberis (*Pao Jiang*), 20g, Folium Photinae Serrulatae (*Shi Nan Ye*), 30g, Radix Salviae Miltiorrhizae (*Dan Shen*), 50g, Radix Ledebouriellae Sesloidis (*Fang Feng*), 30g, Rhizoma Atractylodis Macrocephalae (*Bai Zhu*), 50g, Cortex Radicis Lycii (*Di Gu Pi*), 50g, Rhizoma Ligustici Wallichii (*Chuan Xiong*), 30g, prepared Radix Rehmanniae (*Shu Di*), 40g, Radix Achyranthis Bidentatae (*Niu Xi*), 40g, Fructus Lycii Chinensis (*Gou Qi Zi*), 30g, Radix Gentianae Macrophyllae (*Qin Jiao*), 40g

Method of preparation: Grind the above 15 medicinals into a fine powder and place in a large jar. Soak in 4 *jin* of mellow wine and seal the lid. After 8 days, open the lid, remove the dregs, and decant.

Method of administration: Take 1-2 small teacups warm before meals 3 times per day.

Jia Pi Dan Shen Jiu (Acanthopanax & Salvia Wine)

Functions: Quickens the blood and opens the vessels, strengthens the sinews and disinhibits the joints

Mainly treats: Chilly pain of the joints, ashen white facial color, difficulty bending and flexing the hands and feet, twisting pain in the center of the abdomen

Ingredients: Cortex Radicis Acanthopanacis (*Wu Jia Pi*), 150g, Fructus Citri Seu Ponciri (*Zhi Qiao*), 60g, Radix Salviae Miltiorrhizae (*Dan Shen*), 90g, Cortex Cinnamomi (*Rou Gui*), 30g, stir-fried Radix Angelicae Sinensis (*Dang Gui*), 30g, mix-fried Radix Glycyrrhizae (*Zhi Gan Cao*), 30g, Radix Praeparatus Aconiti Carmichaeli (*Zhi Fu Zi*), 10g, Fructus Zanthoxyli Bungeani (*Shu Jiao*), 30g, Cortex Dictamni Dasycarpi (*Bai Xian Pi*), 30g, Semen Coicis Lachryma-jobi (*Yi Yi Ren*), 15g, Semen Cannabis Sativae (*Huo Ma Ren*), 60g, Caulis Akebiae Mutong (*Mu Tong*), 30g, Rhizoma Ligustici Wallichii (*Chuan Xiong*), 10g, dry Rhizoma Zingiberis (*Gan Jiang*), 10g

Method of preparation: Soak the above 14 medicinals in 3.5 *jin* of white alcohol. Allow to tincture for 4 days in the spring and summer and for 6 days in the fall and winter. Then open the lid, remove the dregs, and store for use.

Method of administration: Take 10-20ml each time warm on an empty stomach. One may increase this dose to 20-30ml per time. When the condition is cured, stop taking.

Ba Ji Tian Jiu (Morinda Wine)

Functions: Supplements the kidneys and reinforces yang, quickens the blood and opens the channels, soothes the sinews and disinhibits the joints

Mainly treats: Chilly pain, stasis and binding in the abdominal region, injury due to lifting a heavy object, *bi* pain of the low back and knees, atony of the feet and lack of strength, inhibited joints of the lower limbs, difficulty bending and flexing the four limbs, kidney vacuity impotence

Ingredients: Radix Morindae Officinalis (*Ba Ji Tian*), 18g, Radix Achyranthis Bidentatae (*Niu Xi*), 18g, Herba Dendrobii (*Shi Hu*), 18g, Radix Et Rhizoma Notopterygii (*Qiang Huo*), 27g, Radix Angelicae Sinensis (*Dang Gui*), 27g, raw Rhizoma Zingiberis (*Sheng Jiang*), 27g, Fructus Zanthoxyli Bungeani (*Shu Jiao*), 2g

Method of preparation: Grind the above 7 ingredients into a fine powder and place in a large jar. Soak in 2 *jin* of alcohol and seal the lid. Then place this in a pan of water and boil for a short time. Remove and allow to cool. Then open and decant.

Method of administration: Take 15-20ml warm each time at no fixed schedule.

Niu Xi Fu Fang Jiu (Achyranthes Compound Wine)

Functions: Quickens the blood and opens the network vessels, supplements yang and strengthens the bones

Ingredients: Herba Dendrobii (*Shi Hu*), 60g, Cortex Eucommiae Ulmoidis (*Du Zhong*), 60g, Radix Salviae Miltiorrhizae (*Dan Shen*), 60g, Radix Rehmanniae (*Sheng Di*), 60g, Radix Achyranthis Bidentatae (*Niu Xi*), 120g

Mainly treats: Kidney vacuity low back pain, inhibited joints, aching and pain of the sinews and bones

Method of preparation: Grind the above five ingredients in a pestle and place in a large jar. Soak in 3 *jin* of alcohol and seal the lid. Open after 7 days and decant.

Method of administration: Take 1 small teacup each time warm before meals

Yi Ren Shi Hu Jiu (Coix & Dendrobium Wine)

Functions: Supplements vacuity and eliminates wind, quickens the blood and opens the network vessels

Mainly treats: Aching and pain of the low back and knees, swelling and fullness of the legs, difficulty walking and moving about, numbness in the four extremities, bodily vacuity and lack of strength, cold pain in the abdomen

Ingredients: Herba Dendrobii (*Shi Hu*), 20g, Radix Salviae Miltior-rhizae (*Dan Shen*), 25g, Cortex Cinnamomi (*Rou Gui*), 15g, Radix Praeparatus Aconiti Carmichaeli (*Zhi Fu Zi*), 20g, Rhizoma Ligustici Wallichii (*Chuan Xiong*), 20g, blast-fried Rhizoma Zingiberis (*Pao Jiang*), 20g, Cortex Radicis Acanthopanacis (*Wu Jia Pi*), 25g, Radix Angelicae Pubescentis (*Du Huo*), 20g, Radix Achyranthis Bidentatae (*Niu Xi*), 20g, Semen Coicis Lachryma-jobi (*Yi Yi Ren*), 100g, Cortex Eucommiae Ulmoidis (*Du Zhong*), 20g, Radix Gentianae Macrophyl-lae (*Qin Jiao*), 20g, Fructus Corni Officinalis (*Shan Zhu Yu*), 25g, Pericarpium Citri Reticulatae (*Chen Pi*), 20g, Radix Astragali Membranacei (*Huang Qi*), 20g, Radix Peucedani (*Bai Qian*), 20g, Caulis Et Folium Skimmiae Reevesianae (*Yin Yu*), 25g, Radix Angelicae Sinensis (*Dang Gui*), 20g, Pulvis Stalactiti (*Zhong Ru Fen*), 40g, Fructus Zanthoxyli (*Shu Jiao*), 20g

Method of preparation: Grind the above 20 medicinals into a fine powder and place in a large jar. Soak in 3 *jin* of alcohol and seal the lid. Open after 4 nights and decant.

Method of administration: Take 1 small teacup warm each time before meals.

Bi Xie Fu Zi Jiu (Dioscorea & Aconite Wine)

Functions: Warms yang and boosts the kidneys, strengthens the low back and knees

Mainly treats: Low back pain, soreness, pain, and contracture and spasm of the sinews and vessels of the foot and knee

Ingredients: Rhizoma Dioscoreae Hypoglaucae (*Bi Xie*), 50g, Radix Praeparatus Aconiti Carmichaeli (*Zhi Fu Zi*), 50g, Rhizoma Cibotii Barometsis (*Gou Ji*), 30g, Cortex Eucommiae Ulmoidis (*Du Zhong*), 30g, Radix Et Rhizoma Notopterygii (*Qiang Huo*), 30g, Cortex Cinnamomi (*Rou Gui*), 30g, Radix Achyranthis Bidentatae (*Niu Xi*), 50g, Ramus Loranthi Seu Visci (*Sang Ji Sheng*), 40g

Method of preparation: Pestle the above 8 ingredients and place in a large jar. Soak in 3 *jin* of alcohol and seal the lid. After 7 days, open and remove the dregs.

Method of administration: Take 1 teacup 3 times per day warm and on an empty stomach.

Di Gu Pi (Cortex Lycii Wine)

Functions: Disinhibits dampness and dispels wind, supplements the liver and boosts the kidneys

Mainly treats: Wind dampness pain of the low back, abnormal vaginal discharge in women, polyuria, turbid urine

Ingredients: Mix-fried Rhizoma Dioscoreae Hypoglaucae (*Zhi Bi Xie*), 50g, Cortex Radicis Lycii (*Di Gu Pi*), 90g, mix-fried Cortex Eucommiae Ulmoidis (*Zhi Du Zhong*), 50g

Method of preparation: Grind the above 3 medicinals into a fine powder and place in a large jar. Soak in 2 *jin* of alcohol and seal the lid. Place this jar in a pan of water and bring to a boil. Then remove the jar and allow to cool. Open, remove the dregs, and store for use.

Method of administration: There is no set time or amount. It is normal to get slightly tipsy on this formula.

Bi Xie Jiu (Dioscorea Hypoglauca Wine)

Functions: Dispels wind dampness, secures the kidney qi

Mainly treats: Wind dampness *bi* pain, impotence and urinary incontinence

Ingredients: Rhizoma Dioscoreae Hypoglaucae (*Bi Xie*), 30g, Radix Ledebouriellae Sesloidis (*Fang Feng*), 15g, Semen Cuscutae (*Tu Si Zi*), 15g, Cortex Eucommiae Ulmoidis (*Du Zhong*), 15g, Radix Astragali Membranacei (*Huang Qi*), 15g, Flos Chrysanthemi Morifolii (*Ju Hua*), 15g, Radix Praeparatus Aconiti Carmichaeli (*Zhi Fu Zi*), 15g, Herba Dendrobii (*Shi Hu*), raw Radix Rehmanniae (*Sheng Di*), 15g, Cortex Radicis Lycii (*Di Gu Pi*), 15g, Radix Dipsaci (*Xu Duan*), 15g, Pyritum (*Zi Ran Tong*), 15g, Folium Photiniae Serrulatae (*Shi Nan Ye*), 15g, Herba Cistanchis (*Rou Cong Rong*), 15g, Fructus Zanthoxyli Bungeani (*Shu Jiao*), 15g

Method of preparation: Grind the above 15 ingredients in a pestle until they are the size of a large bean. Then place them in a large jar.

Soak in 2 *jin* of alcohol. After 14 days, remove the dregs and store for use.

Method of administration: Take 1-2 teacups each time on an empty stomach.

Note: When 1 *jin* of alcohol has been drunk, add another *jin*. The strength of the medicinals will be milder, but the person's condition should, by this time, be better. This can be done 3 times.

Hei Dou Bu Shen Jiu (Black Soybean Supplement the Kidneys Wine)

Functions: Supplements the kidneys and reinforces yang, dispels wind and dampness

Mainly treats: Kidney vacuity low back pain, swelling and pain of the feet and lower legs, physical vacuity weakness

Ingredients: Cooked Semen Glycinis Hispidae (*Hei Dou*), 120g, Cortex Eucommiae Ulmoidis (*Du Zhong*), 40g, prepared Radix Rehmanniae (*Shu Di*), 60g, Fructus Lycii Chinensis (*Gou Qi Zi*), 40g, Radix Et Rhizoma Notopterygii (*Qiang Huo*), 20g, Radix Achyranthis Bidentatae (*Niu Xi*), 30g, Herba Epimedii (*Xian Ling Pi*), 30g, Radix Angelicae Sinensis (*Dang Gui*), 30g, Herba Dendrobii (*Shi Hu*), 20g, Radix Praeparatus Aconiti Carmichaeli (*Zhi Fu Zi*), 30g, Caulis Et Folium Skimmiae Reevesianae (*Yin Yu*), 30g, Sclerotium Poriae Cocos (*Fu Ling*), 30g, Radix Ledebouriellae Sesloidis (*Fang Feng*), 20g, Fructus Zanthoxyli Bungeani (*Chuan Jiao*), 30g, Rhizoma Ligustici Wallichii (*Chuan Xiong*), 20g, Rhizoma Atractylodis Macrocephalae (*Bai Zhu*), 30g, Cortex Radicis Acanthopanacis (*Wu Jia Pi*), 30g, Semen Zizyphi Spinosae (*Suan Zao Ren*), 30g, Cortex Cinnamomi (*Rou Gui*), 20g

Method of preparation: Pestle the above ingredients and then place them in a large jar. Soak in 4 *jin* of alcohol and seal the lid. After 10 days, open, remove the dregs, and store for use.

Method of administration: Take 1 medium teacup each time warm before meals.

Wu Wei Zi Jiu (Schizandra Wine)

Functions: Regulates the qi and harmonizes the blood, tracks down wind and dispels evils

Mainly treats: Heaviness of the body, numbness and insensitivity of the muscles and flesh

Ingredients: Fructus Schizandrae Chinensis (*Wu Wei Zi*), 9g, Radix Ledebouriellae Sesloidis (*Fang Feng*), 9g, Fructus Lycii Chinensis (*Gou Qi Zi*), 9g, Radix Achyranthis Bidentatae (*Niu Xi*), 9g, Cortex Radicis Moutan (*Dan Pi*), 9g, Herba Cistanchis (*Rou Cong Rong*), 9g, Radix Scutellariae Baicalensis (*Huang Qin*), 9g, Rhizoma Atractylodis Macrocephalae (*Bai Zhu*), 9g, Radix Salviae Miltiorrhizae (*Dan Shen*), 9g, Radix Angelicae Sinensis (*Dang Gui*), 9g, stir-fried Fructus Citri Seu Ponciri (*Zhi Qiao*), 9g, mix-fried Radix Glycyrrhizae (*Zhi Gan Cao*), 9g, Cortex Magnoliae Officinalis (*Hou Po*), 9g, Cortex Radicis Acanthopanacis (*Wu Jia Pi*), 9g, Rhizoma Alismatis (*Ze Xie*), 9g, Rhizoma Anemarrhenae (*Zhi Mu*), 9g, Herba Cum Radice Asari (*Xi Xin*), 9g, stir-fried Radix Angelicae (*Bai Zhi*), 9g, Cortex Cinnamomi (*Rou Gui*), 9g

Method of preparation: Pestle the above 19 medicinals until they are the size of large beans and then place them in a large jar. Soak in 2 *jin* of alcohol and seal the lid. After 7 days, open the lid and remove the dregs. Then store for use.

107

Method of administration: Take 15ml each time morning and evening on an empty stomach. One may increase the dose to 20-30ml and even to as much as 40ml.

Shi Nan Fang Feng Jiu (Photinia & Ledebouriella Wine)

Functions: Warms the center and stops pain, eliminates wind dampness, quickens the blood vessels, strengthens the sinews and bones

Mainly treats: Hemiplegia, difficulty stretching the sinews and vessels, inability to bend and flex the lower and upper back, chilly pain in the abdomen

Ingredients: Radix Angelicae Pubescentis (*Du Huo*), 40g, Folium Photiniae Serrulatae (*Shi Nan Ye*), 40g, Radix Ledebouriellae Sesloidis (*Fang Feng*), 30g, Caulis Et Folium Skimmiae Reevesianae (*Yin Yu*), 18g, Radix Praeparatus Aconiti Carmichaeli (*Zhi Fu Zi*), 18g, Radix Aconiti (*Chuan Wu Tou*), 18g, Cortex Cinnamomi (*Rou Gui*), 18g, Radix Achyranthis Bidentatae (*Niu Xi*), 12g

Method of preparation: Grind the above 8 ingredients into a fine powder and place in a large jar. Soak in 3 *jin* of alcohol and seal the lid. Open the lid after 7 days, remove the dregs, and store for use.

Method of administration: Take 1 small teacup warm as often as one wishes.

6

Wines for Dispelling Wind

In Chinese medicine, rheumatic conditions are referred to as *feng shi* or wind dampness. The formulas in this chapter treat such rheumatic joint pain. However, the reader will see that the wines in this chapter are not very different from those in the preceding chapter. They not only contain medicinals which eliminate *bi* pain but also qi and blood, yin and yang supplements. Thus, like the formulas in the preceding chapter, they are especially appropriate for treating older patients and for treating the sequelae of wind stroke.

Mi Chuan Yao Jiu (Secret Transmission Wine)

Functions: Dispels wind, quickens the blood, stops pain, supplements the kidneys

Mainly treats: Paralysis, foot pain, hand and foot numbness and itching

Ingredients: Radix Angelicae Sinensis (*Dang Gui*), 30g, stir-fried Radix Albus Paeoniae Lactiflorae (*Bai Shao*), 30g, raw Radix Rehmanniae (*Sheng Di*), 30g, Radix Achyranthis Bidentatae (*Niu Xi*), 30g, Radix Gentianae Macrophyllae (*Qin Jiao*), 30g, Fructus Chaenomelis Lagenariae (*Mu Gua*), 30g, salt stir-fried Cortex Phellodendri (*Huang Bai*), 30g, ginger stir-fried Cortex Eucommiae Ulmoidis (*Du Zhong*), 30g, Radix Ledebouriellae Sesloidis (*Fang Feng*), 30g, Pericarpium Citri Reticulatae (*Chen Pi*), 30g, Rhizoma Ligustici Wallichii (*Chuan Xiong*), 25g, Radix Et Rhizoma Notopterygii (*Qiang*

Huo), 25g, Radix Angelicae Pubescentis (*Du Huo*), 25g, Radix Angelicae (*Bai Zhi*), 30g, Semen Arecae Catechu (*Bing Lang*), 18g, Cortex Cinnamomi (*Rou Gui*), 10g, mix-fried Radix Glycyrrhizae (*Zhi Gan Cao*), 10g, Nodus Pini (*Fei Song Jie*), 15g

Method of preparation: Place the above 18 ingredients in a large jar and soak in 3 *jin* of alcohol. Then place this jar in a pan of water and boil for 1 hour. Remove the dregs and store for use.

Method of administration: Take whatever amount one wishes each morning and evening.

Pai Jiu Feng (Expel Wind Wine)

Functions: Scatters wind and dispels dampness, resolves tetany and stops pain

Mainly treats: Wind, cold, damp *bi*, aching and pain of the joints of the entire body, chaotic speech, vexation and oppression of the heart and diaphragm, cramping of the four limbs, soreness and pain of the hands and feet

Ingredients: Radix Ledebouriellae Sesloidis (*Fang Feng*), 30g, Rhizoma Cimicifugae (*Sheng Ma*), 30g, Cortex Cinnamomi (*Rou Gui*), 30g, Radix Angelicae Pubescentis (*Du Huo*), Radix Praeparatus Aconiti Carmichaeli (*Zhi Fu Zi*), 30g, Radix Et Rhizoma Notopterygii (*Qiang Huo*), 30g

Method of preparation: Grind the above 6 medicinals into a fine powder and soak in 3 *jin* of mellow wine. After 5 days, open and decant.

Method of administration: Take 20ml each time, 2 times per day.

110

Huang Qi Jiu (Astragalus Wine)

Functions: Dispels wind and scatters cold, warms the kidneys and boosts the qi

Mainly treats: Wind damp *bi* pain, paralysis of the four limbs

Ingredients: Radix Astragali Membranacei (*Huang Qi*), 90g, Radix Angelicae Pubescentis (*Du Huo*), 90g, Radix Ledebouriellae Sesloidis (*Fang Feng*), 90g, mix-fried Radix Glycyrrhizae (*Zhi Gan Cao*), 90g, Fructus Zanthoxyli Bungeani (*Shu Jiao*), 90g, Radix Praeparatus Aconiti Carmichaeli (*Zhi Fu Zi*), 90g, Rhizoma Atractylodis Macrocephalae (*Bai Zhu*), 90g, Radix Achyranthis Bidentatae (*Niu Xi*), 90g, Rhizoma Ligustici Wallichii (*Chuan Xiong*), 90g, Herba Cum Radice Asari (*Xi Xin*), 90g, blast-fried dry Rhizoma Zingiberis (*Pao Gan Jiang*), 100g, Fructus Corni Officinalis (*Shan Zhu Yu*), 75g, Radix Et Rhizoma Rhei (*Da Huang*), 30g, Radix Angelicae Sinensis (*Dang Gui*), 75g, Cortex Cinnamomi (*Rou Gui*), 75g, Radix Puerariae Lobatae (*Ge Gen*), 60g, Radix Gentianae Macrophyllae (*Qin Jiao*), 60g, processed Radix Aconiti (*Zhi Chuan Wu*), 60g

Method of preparation: Grind the above medicinals into powder and place in a large jar. Soak in 4 *jin* of white alcohol and seal the lid. Allow to tincture for 5 days in the spring and summer and for 7 days in the winter and fall. then open the lid, remove the dregs, and store for use.

Method of administration: Take 10-15ml each time warm, 3 times per day. One may increase this dose if necessary.

111

Hai Tong Pi Jiu (Erythrinia Wine)

Functions: Dispels wind dampness

Mainly treats: Wind damp *bi* pain, aching and pain of the joints and lack of strength, feebleness and weakness of the lower legs and knees

Ingredients: Cortex Erythriniae Variegatae (*Hai Tong Pi*), 60g, Radix Achyranthis Bidentatae (*Niu Xi*), 60g, Fructus Citri Seu Ponciri (*Zhi Qiao*), 60g, Cortex Eucommiae Ulmoidis (*Du Zhong*), 60g, Radix Ledebouriellae Sesloidis (*Fang Feng*), 60g, Radix Angelicae Pubescentis (*Du Huo*), 60g, Cortex Radicis Acanthopanacis (*Wu Jia Pi*), 60g, raw Radix Rehmanniae (*Sheng Di*), 70g, Rhizoma Atractylodis Macrocephalae (*Bai Zhu*), 40g, Semen Coicis Lachryma-jobi (*Yi Yi Ren*), 30g

Method of preparation: Grind the above 10 medicinals into a fine powder and place in a large jar. Soak in 4 *jin* of alcohol. After 10 days, open the lid and decant.

Method of administration: Take 10-15ml warm each time, 3 times per day.

Rou Gui Huang Qi Jiu (Cinnamon & Astragalus Wine)

Functions: Warms the middle and scatters cold, dispels wind dampness, stops pain

Mainly treats: Spleen vacuity, fear of cold of the limbs and body, fatigue, lack of strength of the four limbs, joint aching and pain, no desire for food and drink

Ingredients: Radix Astragali Membranacei (*Huang Qi*), 90g, Cortex Cinnamomi (*Rou Gui*), 90g, Radix Morindae Officinalis (*Ba Ji Tian*), 90g, Herba Dendrobii (*Shi Hu*), 90g, Rhizoma Alismatis (*Ze Xie*), 90g, Sclerotium Poriae Cocos (*Fu Ling*), 90g, Rhizoma Aconiti Coreani Seu Typhonii Gigantei (*Bai Fu Zi*), 90g, dry Rhizoma Zingiberis (*Gan Jiang*), 80g, Fructus Zanthoxyli Bungeani (*Shu Jiao*), 90g, Radix Ledebouriellae Sesloidis (*Fang Feng*), 30g, Radix Angelicae Pubescentis (*Du Huo*), 30g, Radix Codonopsis Pilosulae (*Dang Shen*), 30g, Radix Albus Paeoniae Lactiflorae (*Bai Shao*), 30g, Radix Praeparatus Aconiti Carmichaeli (*Zhi Fu Zi*), 30g, processed Radix Aconiti (*Zhi Chuan Wu*), 30g, Caulis Et Folium Skimmiae Reevesianae (*Yin Yu*), 30g, Rhizoma Pinelliae Ternatae (*Ban Xia*), 30g, Herba Cum Radice Asari (*Xi Xin*), 30g, Rhizoma Atractylodis Macrocephalae (*Bai Zhu*), 30g, mix-fried Radix Glycyrrhizae (*Zhi Gan Cao*), 30g, Radix Trichosanthis Kirlowii (*Tian Hua Fen*), 30g, Fructus Corni Officinalis (*Shan Zhu Yu*), 30g

Method of preparation: Grind the above 22 medicinals into a fine powder and place them in a large jar. Soak in 4 *jin* of clear alcohol and seal the lid. Allow to tincture for 7 days in the fall and winter and for 3 days in the spring and summer. Then open, remove the dregs, and store for use.

Method of administration: Begin by taking 30ml and then increase the dosage if necessary. This should produce a slight numbness or tingling which is a good sign.

Quan Xie Jiu (Scorpion Wine)

Functions: Dispels wind and opens the network vessels, transforms phlegm and stops tetany

Mainly treats: Wind stroke, deviation of the eyes and mouth

Ingredients: Rhizoma Aconiti Coreani Seu Typhonii Gigantei (*Bai Fu Zi*), 30g, Bombyx Batryticatus (*Jiang Can*), 30g, Buthus Martensus (*Quan Xie*), 30g

Method of preparation: Grind the above 3 ingredients into a fine powder and place in a large jar. Soak in 1/2 *jin* of mellow wine. After 3 nights, open, remove the dregs, and store for use.

Method of administration: Take 10ml each time at no fixed schedule. It is common to feel the power of the alcohol.

Hei Dou Jiu (Black Soybean Wine)

Functions: Nourishes and quickens the blood, extinguishes wind

Mainly treats: Numbness and pain in the joints, wind damp pain, blood vacuity

Ingredients: Stir-fried Semen Glycinis Hispidae (*Hei Dou*), 500g

Method of preparation: Place the black soybeans in a large jar and soak in 500ml of rice wine. Place this jar in a large pan of water and bring to a boil several times. Allow to cool, remove the dregs, and store for use.

Method of administration: Drink 1 teacup, 2 times per day.

Hei Dou Qiang Huo Jiu (Black Soybean & Notopterygium Wine)

Functions: Resolves the exterior and tracks down wind, overcomes dampness and stops pain

Mainly treats: Wind stroke and aphasia, contracture of the four limbs

Ingredients: Radix Et Rhizoma Notopterygii (*Qiang Huo*), 15g, Radix Ledebouriellae Sesloidis (*Fang Feng*), 10g, stir-fried Semen Glycinis Hispidae (*Hei Dou*), 30g

Method of preparation: Grind the above 3 ingredients into a fine powder. Soak in 200ml of yellow (*i.e.*, rice) wine. Place over a fire and bring to a boil. Then remove the dregs and administer warm.

Method of administration: Divide into two doses and administer by pouring into the patient's mouth.

Du Huo Qiang Huo Jiu (Angelica Pubescens & Notopterygium Wine)

Functions: Dispels wind, stops tetany, eliminates dampness

Mainly treats: The onset of wind stroke, opisthotonos and upper back soreness and pain

Ingredients: Radix Et Rhizoma Notopterygii (*Qiang Huo*), 15g, Rhizoma Ligustici Wallichii (*Chuan Xiong*), 15g, stir-fried & ground Semen Cannabis Sativae (*Huo Ma Ren*), 30g, Semen Glycinis Hispidae (*Hei Dou*), 30g, Radix Angelicae Pubescentis (*Du Huo*), 15g

Method of preparation: Place the Notopterygium, Ligusticum, Cannabis, and Angelica Pubescens in a large jar and soak in 4 *jin* of rice wine for 3 days in the spring and summer and for 7 days in the fall and winter. Then place this jar in a large pan of water and bring to a boil 10 times. Next stir-fry the Black Soybeans and add them to the wine while still hot. Allow to cool and remove the dregs.

115

Method of administration: Take 1-2 small teacups each morning, noon, and night.

Du Huo Shen Fu Jiu (Angelica Pubescens, Codonopsis & Aconite Wine)

Functions: Scatters cold and dispels dampness, warms the middle and stops pain

Mainly treats: Low back and lower leg swelling and pain, inversion counterflow of the four limbs (*i.e.*, chilling), chilly pain in the lower abdomen, bodily vacuity weakness

Ingredients: Radix Angelicae Pubescentis (*Du Huo*), 35g, Radix Praeparatus Aconiti Carmichaeli (*Zhi Fu Zi*), 35g, Radix Codonopsis Pilosulae (*Dang Shen*), 20g

Method of preparation: Grind the above 3 medicinals into a fine powder and place in a large jar. Soak in 1 *jin* of alcohol and seal the lid. Allow to tincture for 5 days in the spring and summer and for 7 days in the fall and winter.

Method of administration: Each time take as much as one desires. It is common or normal to feel the alcohol qi (*i.e.*, to feel a little tipsy).

Dang Gui Song Ye Jiu (Dang Gui & Pine Needle Wine)

Functions: Scatters wind, quickens the blood, and dispels cold

Mainly treats: Aching and pain of the joints, inability to use the limbs

Ingredients: Fresh Folium Pini (*Xin Song Ye*), 2 *jin*, Radix Angelicae Sinensis (*Dang Gui*), 150g

Method of preparation: Place these above 2 ingredients in a large jar and soak in 5 *jin* of clear alcohol. After 41 days open, remove the dregs, and store for use.

Method of administration: Use as one pleases in terms of amount and times.

Xi Xin Du Huo Jiu (Asarum & Angelica Pubescens Wine)

Functions: Dispels wind, stops pain, disperses swelling

Mainly treats: Tooth and gum swelling and pain

Ingredients: Radix Angelicae Pubescentis (*Du Huo*), 15g, Radix Ledebouriellae Sesloidis (*Fang Feng*), 15g, Herba Illicii Lanceolati (*Mang Cao*), 15g, Herba Cum Radice Asari (*Xi Xin*), 15g, Radix Praeparatus Aconiti Carmichaeli (*Zhi Fu Zi*), 6g

Method of preparation: Grind the above 5 medicinals into a fine powder and place in a large jar. Soak in 1/2 *jin* of alcohol. Place this jar in a large pot of water and bring to a boil 10 times. Then remove the dregs and store for use.

Method of administration: Drink hot. Stop taking when cured.

Du Huo Shi Hu Jiu (Angelica Pubescens & Dendrobium Wine)

Functions: Dispels wind and eliminates dampness, supplements vacuity and quickens the blood

Mainly treats: Invasion by wind dampness, low back and lower leg soreness and pain, difficulty walking and moving about, dizziness and vertigo

Ingredients: Radix Angelicae Pubescentis (*Du Huo*), 40g, blast-fried Rhizoma Zingiberis (*Pao Jiang*), 20g, Herba Dendrobii (*Shi Hu*), 30g, Radix Achyranthis Bidentatae (*Niu Xi*), 30g, Radix Salviae Miltiorrhizae (*Dan Shen*), 30g, Rhizoma Dioscoreae Hypoglaucae (*Bi Xie*), 30g, Radix Praeparatus Aconiti Carmichaeli (*Zhi Fu Zi*), 30g, Sclerotium Rubrum Poriae Cocos (*Chi Fu Ling*), 30g, Radix Ledebouriellae Sesloidis (*Fang Feng*), 20g, Semen Coicis Lachryma-jobi (*Yi Yi Ren*), 40g, Fructus Corni Officinalis (*Shan Zhu Yu*), 30g, Cortex Cinnamomi (*Rou Gui*), 20g, Rhizoma Atractylodis Macrocephalae (*Bai Zhu*), 20g, Rhizoma Ligustici Wallichii (*Chuan Xiong*), 20g, Radix Gentianae Macrophyllae (*Qin Jiao*), 30g, Radix Angelicae Sinensis (*Dang Gui*), 20g, Radix Panacis Ginseng (*Ren Shen*), 20g, Flos Chrysanthemi Morifolii (*Gan Ju Hua*), 20g, Radix Rehmanniae (*Sheng Di*)

Method of preparation: Pestle the above 19 ingredients into pieces and place in a large jar. Soak in 5 *jin* of alcohol. After 7 days, open and remove the dregs. Store for use.

Method of administration: Take a suitable amount warm each time before meals.

118

Du Huo Niu Xi Jiu (Angelica Pubescens & Achyranthes Wine)

Functions: Warms the channels and harmonizes the blood, eliminates dampness and stops pain

Mainly treats: Wind stroke with hemiplegia, aching and pain of the joints of the bones

Ingredients: Radix Angelicae Pubescentis (*Du Huo*), 30g, Cortex Cinnamomi (*Rou Gui*), 30g, Radix Ledebouriellae Sesloidis (*Fang Feng*), 30g, Radix Praeparatus Aconiti Carmichaeli (*Zhi Fu Zi*), 30g, Semen Cannabis Sativae (*Huo Ma Ren*), stir-fried till fragrant, 50g, Radix Achyranthis Bidentatae (*Niu Xi*), 30g, Fructus Zanthoxyli Bungeani (*Chuan Jiao*), 50g

Method of preparation: Grind the above ingredients into a fine powder and place in a large jar. Soak in 3 *jin* of alcohol and seal the lid. After 3 days, open, remove the dregs, and store for use.

Method of administration: Each day take 1 medium teacup warm before meals. Healing should not take more than 2-3 formulas (*i.e.*, packets of herbs).

Du Huo Dang Gui Jiu (Angelica Pubescens & *Dang Gui* Wine)

Functions: Dispels wind dampness, soothes the joints

Mainly treats: Wind damp low back and lower leg aching and pain

Ingredients: Radix Angelicae Pubescentis (*Du Huo*), 30g, Cortex Eucommiae Ulmoidis (*Du Zhong*), 30g, Radix Angelicae Sinensis

(*Dang Gui*), 30g, Rhizoma Ligustici Wallichii (*Chuan Xiong*), 30g, prepared Radix Rehmanniae (*Shu Di*), 30g, Radix Salviae Miltiorrhizae (*Dan Shen*), 30g

Method of preparation: Grind the above 6 medicinals into a fine powder and place them in a large jar. Soak in 2 *jin* of good alcohol and seal the lid. Warm by a fire for 1 day and night. Then allow to cool, remove the dregs, and store for use.

Method of administration: There is no set time or amount when drinking this wine. It is normal to feel the alcohol qi.

Zhu Feng Du Huo Jiu (Dispel Wind Angelica Pubescens Wine)

Functions: Dispels wind dampness, stops pain

Mainly treats: Low back and knee soreness and pain, lower leg and foot heaviness, aching, and pain

Ingredients: Radix Angelicae Pubescentis (*Du Huo*), 60g

Method of preparation: Place the above ingredient in 250ml of white alcohol. After 4-5 days, open the lid and remove the dregs. Store for use.

Method of administration: Take 1 small teacup warm each time on an empty stomach, 3 times per day.

Chang Pu Jiu (Acorus Wine)

Functions: Opens the portals and dispels phlegm, scatters wind and dispels dampness, loosens the center and harmonizes the stomach

Mainly treats: Withdrawal and mania, fright epilepsy, confused spirit, delirious speech, ringing in the ears, poor memory, insomnia, inhibition of the joints, counterflow cough with copious phlegm, chest and abdominal distention and oppression, glomus of the venter, lack of hunger, vomiting

Ingredients: Rhizoma Acori Graminei (*Shi Chang Pu*), 120g

Method of preparation: Soak the Acorus in 450ml of alcohol and seal the lid. After 3-5 days, open and remove the dregs. Store for use.

Method of administration: Take 10-20ml on an empty stomach, 3 times per day.

Chan Sha Jiu (Silkworm Wine)

Functions: Dispels wind and eliminates dampness, harmonizes the stomach and transforms turbidity

Mainly treats: Wind damp *bi* pain, itching of the skin, dormant papules, head wind, headache, twisted sinews, vomiting and diarrhea

Ingredients: Stir-fried till yellow Bombyx Batryticatus (*Chan Sha*), 60g

Method of preparation: Place the Silkworms in a large jar and soak in 200ml of mellow alcohol. Seal the lid. After 5 days, open and remove the dregs.

Method of administration: Take 1 small teacup warm each time on an empty stomach, 3 times per day.

Shi Wei Fu Zi Jiu (Ten Flavors Aconite Wine)

Functions: Scatters cold and dispels dampness

Mainly treats: Foot qi leading to weakness and lack of strength of the feet and lower legs, possible numbness, soreness and pain, swelling and distention, fever, vomiting, etc.

Ingredients: Radix Praeparatus Aconiti Carmichaeli (*Zhi Fu Zi*), 30g, Cortex Radicis Acanthopanacis (*Wu Jia Pi*), 20g, Radix Salviae Miltiorrhizae (*Dan Shen*), 30g, Radix Dipsaci (*Xu Duan*), 30g, Radix Achyranthis Bidentatae (*Niu Xi*), 30g, Rhizoma Atractylodis Macrocephalae (*Bai Zhu*), 50g, fresh Rhizoma Zingiberis (*Sheng Jiang*), 50g, Cortex Radicis Mori Albi (*Sang Bai Pi*), 50g, Herba Cum Radice Asari (*Xi Xin*), 25g, Cortex Cinnamomi (*Rou Gui*), 25g

Method of preparation: Grind the above 10 ingredients into a fine powder and wrap them in a cloth bag. Place this in a large jar and soak in 3 *jin* of clear alcohol. Seal the lid. After 5 days in the spring and summer and 7 days in the fall and winter, open, remove the dregs, and store for use.

Method of administration: Take 1 small teacup warm on an empty stomach, 3 times per day.

Shi Hu Fu Zi Jiu (Dendrobium & Aconite Wine)

Functions: Expels wind and eliminates dampness, quickens the blood and transforms stasis, warms the center and scatters cold

122

Mainly treats: Foot and lower leg weakness and lack of strength, aching and pain difficult to bear, inability to move the four limbs, chilly pain within the umbilicus

Ingredients: Radix Praeparatus Aconiti Carmichaeli (*Zhi Fu Zi*), 40g, Herba Dendrobii (*Shi Hu*), 20g, Radix Angelicae Pubescentis (*Du Huo*), 40g, Fructus Perillae Frutescentis (*Zi Su*), 20g, Herba Epimedii (*Xian Ling Pi*), 10g, Radix Ledebouriellae Sesloidis (*Fang Feng*), 10g, Sclerotium Rubrum Poriae Cocos (*Chi Fu Ling*), 10g, Radix Scutellariae Baicalensis (*Huang Qin*), 10g, Radix Stephaniae Tetrandrae (*Fang Ji*), 10g, Cortex Cinnamomi (*Rou Gui*), 10g, Radix Salviae Miltiorrhizae (*Dan Shen*), 10g, Fructus Zanthoxyli Bungeani (*Chuan Jiao*), 10g, Rhizoma Ligustici Wallichii (*Chuan Xiong*), 10g, Herba Cum Radice Asari (*Xi Xin*), 15g, Radix Angelicae Sinensis (*Dang Gui*), 20g, Rhizoma Atractylodis Macrocephalae (*Bai Zhu*), 20g, Radix Clematidis Sinensis (*Wei Ling Xian*), 20g, Semen Coicis Lachrymajobi (*Yi Yi Ren*), 10g, stir-fried Semen Glycinis Hispidae (*Hei Dou*), 300g, Radix Gentianae Macrophyllae (*Qin Jiao*), 20g

Method of preparation: Grind the above ingredients in a mortar with a pestle and then place in a large jar. Soak in 3 *jin* of good alcohol. After 7 days, open, remove the dregs, and store for use.

Method of administration: Take a suitable amount warm before each meal.

Du Huo Fu Zi Jiu (Angelica Pubescens & Aconite Wine)

Functions: Scatters cold and stops pain, dispels dampness and eliminates *bi*

Mainly treats: Swelling and distention of the foot and lower leg, aching, pain, and numbness, contracture and spasm of the sinews and vessels

Ingredients: Radix Praeparatus Aconiti Carmichaeli (*Fu Zi*), 50g, Radix Angelicae Pubescentis (*Du Huo*), 50g

Method of preparation: Grind the above 2 medicinals into a fine powder and place in a large jar. Soak in 1 *jin* of mellow wine. After 5 days, open, remove the dregs, and store for use.

Method of administration: Take 1 small teacup warm before meals, 3 times per day.

Fu Zi Dan Sha Jiu (Aconite & Cinnabar Wine)

Functions: Dispels wind and eliminates dampness, scatters cold and opens the network vessels

Mainly treats: Low back and leg atony and weakness, difficulty walking and moving about, superficial edema of the skin, numbness and insensitivity of the muscles and flesh

Ingredients: Radix Praeparatus Aconiti Carmichaeli (*Zhi Fu Zi*), 25g, Radix Achyranthis Bidentatae (*Niu Xi*), 25g, Cinnabar (*Dan Sha*), 25g, Fructus Corni Officinalis (*Shan Zhu Yu*), 25g, mix-fried Cortex Eucommiae Ulmoidis (*Du Zhong*), 25g, Herba Dendrobii (*Shi Hu*), 25g, Caulis Et Folium Sambucudis Javanicae (*Lu Ying Gen*), 20g, Radix Ledebouriellae Sesloidis (*Fang Feng*), 18g, Fructus Zanthoxyli Bungeani (*Shu Jiao*), 18g, Herba Cum Radice Asari (*Xi Xin*), 18g, Radix Angelicae Pubescentis (*Du Huo*), 18g, Radix Gentianae Macrophyllae (*Qin Jiao*), 18g, Cortex Cinnamomi (*Rou Gui*), 10g, Rhizoma Ligustici Wallichii (*Chuan Xiong*), 18g, Radix Angelicae

Sinensis (*Dang Gui*), 18g, Rhizoma Atractylodis Macrocephalae (*Bai Zhu*), 18g, Caulis Et Folium Skimmiae Reevesianae (*Yin Yu*), 15g, Cortex Radicis Acanthopanacis (*Wu Jia Pi*), 30g, Semen Coicis Lachryma-jobi (*Yi Yi Ren*), 80g, blast-fried dry Rhizoma Zingiberis (*Pao Gan Jiang*), 12g

Method of preparation: Pestle the above ingredients into pieces and wrap in a cloth bag. Soak in 4 *jin* of alcohol and seal the lid. Allow to tincture for 4 nights in the spring and summer and for 7 nights in the fall and winter. Then open the lid and remove the dregs.

Method of administration: There are no fixed times for taking this wine. Begin by taking 10ml and increase to 20ml if necessary. Once healed, stop taking.

Shi Qi Wei Yao Jiu (Seventeen Flavors Herbal Wine)

Functions: Dispels wind, disinhibits dampness, supplements vacuity

Mainly treats: Wind damp *bi* pain, sinew and vessel contracture and spasm, low back and leg weakness and lack of strength, seeing and hearing unclear

Ingredients: Radix Achyranthis Bidentatae (*Niu Xi*), 90g, Quartz (*Bai Shi Ying*), 120g, Magnetitum (*Ci Shi*), 120g, Herba Dendrobii (*Shi Hu*), 90g, Radix Praeparatus Aconiti Carmichaeli (*Zhi Fu Zi*), 90g, Rhizoma Hypoglaucae (*Bi Xie*), 30g, Radix Salviae Miltiorrhizae (*Dan Shen*), 30g, Radix Ledebouriellae Sesloidis (*Fang Feng*), 30g, Fructus Corni Officinalis (*Shan Zhu Yu*), 30g, Radix Astragali Membranacei (*Huang Qi*), 30g, Radix Et Rhizoma Notopterygii (*Qiang Huo*), Cornu Antelopis (*Ling Yang Jiao*), 30g, Semen Zizyphi Spinosae (*Suan Zao Ren*), 30g, Radix Rehmanniae (*Sheng Di*), 60g,

Cortex Cinnamomi (*Rou Gui*), 60g, Sclerotium Poriae Cocos (*Fu Ling*), 60g, Cortex Eucommiae Ulmoidis (*Du Zhong*), 45g

Method of preparation: Grind the above 17 ingredients into a fine powder and place in a large jar. Soak in 7 *jin* of alcohol. After 10 days, open, remove the dregs, and store for use.

Method of administration: Take 1 small teacup warm on an empty stomach morning and evening.

Fu Zi Bai Zhu Jiu (Aconite & Atractylodes Wine)

Functions: Scatters cold and dispels dampness, dispels wind and stops pain, rescues yang and warms the center

Mainly treats: Inversion counterflow (*i.e.*, chill) of the four extremities, numbness and insensitivity of the skin and muscles, low back pain, impotence, weak heart function, chilly pain in the abdominal region, vomiting and chilly diarrhea, aching and pain of the joints

Ingredients: Radix Praeparatus Aconiti Carmichaeli (*Zhi Fu Zi*), 30g, Radix Ledebouriellae Sesloidis (*Fang Feng*), 30g, Radix Et Rhizoma Notopterygii (*Qiang Huo*), 30g, Radix Angelicae Sinensis (*Dang Gui*), 30g, Rhizoma Atractylodis Macrocephalae (*Bai Zhu*), 30g, Cortex Radicis Acanthopanacis (*Wu Jia Pi*), 25g, Rhizoma Ligustici Wallichii (*Chuan Xiong*), 25g, Cortex Cinnamomi (*Rou Gui*), 25g, blast-fried Rhizoma Zingiberis (*Pao Jiang*), 25g

Method of preparation: Pestle the above 9 medicinals and break them up into small pieces. Wrap in a cloth bag and place in a large jar. Soak in 2 *jin* of white alcohol for 5 days in the spring and summer and for 7 days in the fall and winter. Then remove the dregs and store for use.

Method of administration: Take 15-20ml warm each time. It is also all right to take more or less as one desires, but it is not all right to become drunk. Stop taking when a cure has been obtained.

Huang Qi Xu Duan Jiu (Astragalus & Dipsacus Wine)

Functions: Dispels wind dampness, supplements vacuity

Mainly treats: Wind damp *bi* pain, generalized numbness, itching of the skin, sinew and vessel contracture and spasm, inability to use the hands and feet, a weak, indistinct voice

Ingredients: Radix Astragali Membranacei (*Huang Qi*), 30g, Radix Ledebouriellae Sesloidis (*Fang Feng*), 30g, Cortex Cinnamomi (*Rou Gui*), 30g, Rhizoma Gastrodiae Elatae (*Tian Ma*), 30g, Rhizoma Dioscoreae Hypoglaucae (*Bi Xie*), 30g, Radix Albus Paeoniae Lactiflorae (*Bai Shao*), 30g, Radix Angelicae Sinensis (*Dang Gui*), 30g, Pulvis Muscovitum (*i.e.*, Mica, *Yun Mu Fen*), 30g, Rhizoma Atractylodis Macrocephalae (*Bai Zhu*), 30g, Caulis Et Folium Skimmiae Reevesianae (*Yin Yu Ye*), 20g, Radix Saussureae Seu Vladimiriae (*Mu Xiang*), 30g, Herba Epimedii (*Xian Ling Pi*), 30g, Radix Glycyrrhizae (*Gan Cao*), 30g, Radix Dipsaci (*Xu Duan*), 30g

Method of preparation: Grind the above 14 medicinals into a fine powder and place in a large jar. Soak in 5 *jin* of good alcohol. After 7 days, open, remove the dregs, and store for use.

Method of administration: Take 1 teacup warm at no set time.

Zhong Ru Jiu (Stalactite Wine)

Functions: Dispels wind and eliminates dampness, quickens the blood and stops pain .

Mainly treats: Wind damp *bi* pain, weakness of the feet and knees

Ingredients: Stalactitum (*Zhong Ru Shi*), 100g, Radix Salviae Miltiorrhizae (*Dan Shen*), 60g, Herba Dendrobii (*Shi Hu*), 60g, Cortex Eucommiae Ulmoidis (*Du Zhong*), 60g, Tuber Asparagi Cochinensis (*Tian Men Dong*), 60g, Radix Achyranthis Bidentatae (*Niu Xi*), 60g, Radix Ledebouriellae Sesloidis (*Fang Feng*), 60g, Radix Astragali Membranacei (*Huang Qi*), 60g, Rhizoma Ligustici Wallichii (*Chuan Xiong*), 60g, Radix Angelicae Sinensis (*Dang Gui*), 60g, Radix Praeparatus Aconiti Carmichaeli (*Zhi Fu Zi*), 30g, Cortex Cinnamomi (*Rou Gui*), 30g, Radix Gentianae Macrophyllae (*Qin Jiao*), 30g, dry Rhizoma Zingiberis (*Gan Jiang*), 30g, Fructus Corni Officinalis (*Shan Zhu Yu*), 100g, Semen Coicis Lachryma-jobi (*Yi Yi Ren*), 100g

Method of preparation: Grind the above 16 ingredients into a fine powder and place in a large jar. Soak in 5 *jin* of good alcohol. After 3 days, open, remove the dregs, and store for use.

Method of administration: Take 10ml warm each time at no fixed schedule. One can increase the dosage until one feels their lips become numb and tingling.

Fang Feng Bai Zhu Jiu (Ledebouriella & Atractylodes Wine)

Functions: Regulates and harmonizes the qi and blood, tracks down wind and dispels evils

128

Mainly treats: Numbness and insensitivity of the muscles and flesh, generalized heaviness of the body, aching and pain of the joints

Ingredients: Radix Ledebouriellae Sesloidis (*Fang Feng*), 12g, Rhizoma Atractylodis Macrocephalae (*Bai Zhu*), 9g, Fructus Corni Officinalis (*Shan Zhu Yu*), 9g, Radix Praeparatus Aconiti Carmichaeli (*Zhi Fu Zi*), 9g, Magnetitum (*Ci Shi*), 50g, slightly stir-fried Herba Cum Radice Asari (*Xi Xin*), 9g, Radix Angelicae Pubescentis (*Du Huo*), 9g, Radix Gentianae Macrophyllae (*Qin Jiao*), 9g, Caulis Et Folium Skimmiae Reevesianae (*Yin Yu*), 9g, Radix Dioscoreae Oppositae (*Shan Yao*), 9g, stir-fried Semen Pruni Armeniacae (*Xing Ren*), 9g, Radix Morindae Officinalis (*Ba Ji Tian*), 12g, Cortex Cinnamomi (*Rou Gui*), 12g, Herba Ephedrae (*Ma Huang*), 12g, fresh Rhizoma Zingiberis (*Sheng Jiang*), 30g, stir-fried Semen Coicis Lachryma-jobi (*Yi Yi Ren*), 18g, Radix Rehmanniae (*Sheng Di*), 15g

Method of preparation: Grind the above 17 ingredients into a fine powder and wrap them in a cloth bag. Place in a large jar and soak in 2 *jin* of clear alcohol. Seal the lid. After 7 days, open, remove the dregs, and store for use.

Method of administration: Take 20ml warm on an empty stomach morning and evening.

Tong Pi Yi Ren Jiu (Erythrinia & Coix Wine)

Functions: Dispels wind and eliminates dampness, opens the channels and network vessels, kills worms (*i.e.*, parasites)

Mainly treats: Serious low back and knee damp heat pain, blood vessel obstinate *bi* upper arm pain, inability to use the feet and legs, mange

129

Ingredients: Cortex Erythriniae (*Hai Tong Pi*), 60g, Semen Coicis Lachryma-jobi (*Yi Yi Ren*), 60g, Radix Rehmanniae (*Sheng Di*), 100g, Radix Cyathulae (*Chuan Niu Xi*), 30g, Rhizoma Ligustici Wallichii (*Chuan Xiong*), 30g, Radix Et Rhizoma Notopterygii (*Qiang Huo*), 30g, Cortex Radicis Lycii (*Di Gu Pi*), 30g, Cortex Radicis Acantho-panacis (*Wu Jia Pi*), 30g, Radix Glycyrrhizae (*Gan Cao*), 12g

Method of preparation: Grind the above 9 ingredients into a fine powder and place in a large jar. Soak in 3 *jin* of white alcohol and seal the lid. After 7 days in the summer and 10 days in the winter, open, remove the dregs, and store for use.

Method of administration: Take 15-20ml each time on an empty stomach, 3 times per day. It is normal to feel slightly tipsy.

Dang Gui Xi Xin Jiu (Dang Gui & Asarum Wine)

Functions: Tracks down wind and scatters cold, harmonizes the blood and stops pain

Mainly treats: Wind damp *bi* pain, contracture and inability to use the body and limbs

Ingredients: Radix Angelicae Sinensis (*Dang Gui*), 45g, Herba Cum Radice Asari (*Xi Xin*), 45g, Radix Ledebouriellae Sesloidis (*Fang Feng*), 45g, Radix Praeparatus Aconiti Carmichaeli (*Zhi Fu Zi*), 10g, Herba Ephedrae (*Ma Huang*), 35g, Radix Angelicae Pubescentis (*Du Huo*), 90g

Method of preparation: Pestle the above medicinals into small pieces and decoct in 3 *jin* of alcohol down to 2 *jin*. Then remove the dregs and store for use.

Method of administration: Take 10-20ml warm after each meal.

Bai Shi Ying Jiu (Quartz Wine)

Functions: Dispels wind dampness, disinhibits the joints, calms the spirit and improves hearing

Mainly treats: Wind damp natured generalized body aching and pain, swelling and pain of the joints, lack of strength in movement and activity, poor hearing due to kidney viscus vacuity detriment

Ingredients: Quartz (*Bai Shi Ying*), 30g, Magnetitum (*Ci Shi*), 30g

Method of preparation: Grind the above 2 medicinals into a fine powder and place in a large jar. Soak in 1 *jin* of alcohol and seal the lid. After 5-6 days, open, remove the dregs, and store for use.

Method of administration: Take a suitable amount warm at no fixed times.

Cao Wu Jiu (Cao Wu Aconite Wine)

Functions: Dispels wind dampness, harmonizes the blood and stops pain

Mainly treats: Wind damp natured hand and foot aching and pain. It also treats goose foot leprosy in women.

Ingredients: Processed Radix Aconiti (*Zhi Cao Wu*), 20g, Radix Angelicae Sinensis (*Dang Gui*), 70g, Radix Albus Paeoniae Lactiflorae (*Bai Shao*), 70g, Semen Glycinis Hispidae (*Hei Dou*), 70g, Caulis Lonicerae (*Ren Dong Teng*), 90g

131

Method of preparation: First stir-fry and then parboil the Black Soybeans. Next add these and the other 4 ingredients to 3 *jin* of alcohol and allow to tincture to 5 days. Open, remove the dregs, and store for use.

Method of administration: Take a suitable amount warm at no fixed times.

Du Huo Ji Sheng Jiu (Angelica Pubescens & Loranthus Wine)

Functions: Boosts the liver and kidneys, supplements the qi and blood, dispels wind dampness, stops *bi* pain

Mainly treats: Wind, cold, damp *bi*, aching and pain of the joints, low back and knee soreness and pain, numbness of the body and limbs, all worse on rainy, damp days

Ingredients: Radix Angelicae Pubescentis (*Du Huo*), 30g, Ramus Loranthi Seu Visci (*Sang Ji Sheng*), 20g, Radix Gentianae Macrophyllae (*Qin Jiao*), 30g, Radix Ledebouriellae Sesloidis (*Fang Feng*), 20g, Herba Cum Radice Asari (*Xi Xin*), 12g, Radix Angelicae Sinensis (*Dang Gui*), 50g, Radix Albus Paeoniae Lactiflorae (*Bai Shao*), 30g, Rhizoma Ligustici Wallichii (*Chuan Xiong*), 20g, Radix Rehmanniae (*Sheng Di*), 50g, Cortex Eucommiae Ulmoidis (*Du Zhong*), 50g, Radix Achyranthis Bidentatae (*Niu Xi*), 30g, Radix Codonopsis Pilosulae (*Dang Shen*), 30g, Sclerotium Poriae Cocos (*Fu Ling*), 40g, Radix Glycyrrhizae (*Gan Cao*), 15g, Cortex Cinnamomi (*Rou Gui*), 15g

Method of preparation: Break up these 15 ingredients in a mortar and pestle and then place in a large jar. Soak in 3 *jin* of mellow wine and seal the lid. After 14 days, open, remove the dregs, and store for use.

Method of administration: Take a suitable amount each time at no fixed schedule.

Qin Jiao Gui Ling Jiu (Gentiana Macrophylla, Cinnamon & Poria Wine)

Functions: Warms and supplements kidney yang, eliminates dampness and dispels wind

Mainly treats: Vacuity chill of the low back and knees, prolonged sitting on damp earth, wind damp *bi* pain

Ingredients: Radix Gentianae Macrophyllae (*Qin Jiao*), 30g, Radix Achyranthis Bidentatae (*Niu Xi*), 30g, Rhizoma Ligustici Wallichii (*Chuan Xiong*), 30g, Radix Ledebouriellae Sesloidis (*Fang Feng*), 30g, Cortex Cinnamomi (*Rou Gui*), 30g, Radix Angelicae Pubescentis (*Du Huo*), 30g, Sclerotium Poriae Cocos (*Fu Ling*), 30g, Cortex Eucommiae Ulmoidis (*Du Zhong*), 60g, Radix Salviae Miltiorrhizae (*Dan Shen*), 60g, Radix Praeparatus Aconiti Carmichaeli (*Zhi Fu Zi*), 35g, Herba Dendrobii (*Shi Hu*), 35g, blast-fried Rhizoma Zingiberis (*Pao Jiang*), 35g, Tuber Ophiopogonis Japonicae (*Mai Men Dong*), 35g, Cortex Radicis Lycii (*Di Gu Pi*), 35g, Cortex Radicis Acantho-panacis (*Wu Jia Pi*), 60g, Semen Coicis Lachryma-jobi (*Yi Yi Ren*), 30g, stir-fried Semen Cannabis Sativae (*Huo Ma Ren*), 15g

Method of preparation: Grind the above 17 ingredients into a fine powder and place in a large jar. Soak in 4 *jin* of alcohol for 7 days in the spring and fall, for 3 days in the summer, and for 10 days in the winter. Remove the dregs and store for use.

Method of administration: Take 1-2 teacups warm on an empty stomach, 3 times per day.

Hei Dou Bai Zhi Jiu (Black Soybean & Angelica Wine)

Functions: Disinhibits water and disperses swelling, nourishes the blood and levels the liver, transforms dampness and eliminates *bi*

Mainly treats: Foot qi, *bi*, and weakness, dizziness and vertigo, sinew spasm, inhibited urination

Ingredients: Stir-fried Semen Glycinis Hispidae (*Hei Dou*), 250g, Radix Angelicae (*Bai Zhi*), 30g, Semen Coicis Lachryma-jobi (*Yi Yi Ren*), 60g

Method of preparation: Grind the above 3 ingredients into a fine powder and place in a large jar. Soak in 3 *jin* of yellow (*i.e.,* rice) wine and seal the lid. After 3 nights, open, remove the dregs, and store for use.

Method of administration: Each day, drink a suitable amount at appropriate times. It is common to feel the power of the alcohol.

Hei Dou Dan Shen Jiu (Black Soybean & Salvia Wine)

Functions: Quickens the blood and dispels stasis, disinhibits dampness and eliminates *bi*

Mainly treats: Wind stroke paralysis of the hands and feet

Ingredients: Semen Glycinis Hispidae (*Hei Dou*), 250g, Radix Salviae Miltiorrhizae (*Dan Shen*), 150g

Method of preparation: Pestle these two medicinals and place in a large jar. Soak in 4 *jin* of yellow (*i.e.*, rice) wine and seal the lid. Place over a fire and bring to a boil. Reduce the alcohol by half. Then remove the dregs and decant.

Method of administration: Take 1-2 teacups each time, morning, noon, and night.

Bai Hua She Jiu (White Flower Snake Wine)

Functions: Dispels wind dampness

Mainly treats: Contracture and spasm of the sinews and vessels, hemiplegia

Ingredients: Agkistrodon Seu Bungarus (*Bai Hua She*), 1 strip

Method of preparation: Grind up into pieces and soak in 500g of white alcohol for 15 days.

Method of administration: Take 15ml each evening.

Fu Fang Bai She Jiu (Compound White Snake Wine)

Functions: Dispels wind dampness

Mainly treats: Low back and leg aching and pain, difficulty walking and moving about, itching and pain of the skin

Ingredients: Agkistrodon Seu Bungarus (*Bai Hua She*), 1 strip, Radix Angelicae Sinensis (*Dang Gui*), 30g, Rhizoma Ligustici Wallichii (*Chuan Xiong*), 30g, Radix Praeparatus Aconiti Carmichaeli

(*Zhi Fu Zi*), 40g, Cortex Cinnamomi (*Rou Gui*), 40g, prepared Radix Rehmanniae (*Shu Di*), 40g, Fructus Corni Officinalis (*Shan Zhu Yu*), 40g, Rhizoma Dioscoreae Hypoglaucae (*Bi Xie*), 40g, Herba Dendrobii (*Shi Hu*), 40g, Herba Cum Radice Asari (*Xi Xin*), 40g, Radix Astragali Membranacei (*Huang Qi*), 40g, Rhizoma Gastrodiae Elatae (*Tian Ma*), 40g, Radix Angelicae Pubescentis (*Du Huo*), 60g, Fructus Citri Seu Ponciri (*Zhi Qiao*), 25g, Herba Cistanchis (*Rou Cong Rong*), 40g

Method of preparation: Grind the above 15 medicinals into a coarse powder and place in a large jar. Soak in 6 *jin* of mellow wine and seal the lid. After 7 days, open, remove the dregs, and store for use.

Method of administration: Take a suitable amount warm at no fixed times. It is common to feel a little tipsy.

Wu Shao She Jiu (Black Stripe Snake Wine)

Functions: Dispels wind and opens the network vessels, combats toxins

Mainly treats: Wind damp *bi* pain, numbness and tingling of the muscles and skin, nodulations of the bones and joints, pediatric palsy

Ingredients: Zaocys Dhumnades (*Wu Shao She*), 1 strip

Method of preparation: Place the Zaocys Dhumandes in a large jar and soak for 3-4 days in good alcohol.

Method of administration: Take 1-2 teacups 3 times per day.

Chuan Xiong Qiang Huo Jiu (Ligusticum & Notopterygium Wine)

Functions: Dispels wind and stops pain, quickens the blood and opens the network vessels

Mainly treats: Heat toxins and wind evils resulting in mouth and facial paralysis and hemilateral wind

Ingredients: Rhizoma Ligustici Wallichii (*Chuan Xiong*), 30g, Radix Et Rhizoma Notopterygii (*Qiang Huo*), 30g, Herba Illicii Lanceolati (*Mang Cao*), 20g, Herba Cum Radice Asari (*Xi Xin*), 30g, mix-fried Radix Glycyrrhizae (*Zhi Gan Cao*), 30g, stir-fried Semen Glycinis Hispidae (*Hei Dou*), 60g

Method of preparation: Grind the above 6 medicinals into a fine powder. Then divide into 8 doses. Each time use 1 dose in 100ml of alcohol and decoct down to 50ml.

Method of administration: Each day take 4-5 doses.

Jin Ya Fang Feng Jiu (Pyritum & Ledebouriella Wine)

Functions: Diffuses obstruction and dispels dampness, dispels wind and warms the center

Mainly treats: Wind cold invading the muscles and body, chilly pain of the low back and knees, contracture and spasm of the sinews and bones, inability to use the legs and feet

Ingredients: Pyritum (*Jin Ya Shi, i.e., Zi Ran Tong*), 20g, Herba Cum Radice Asari (*Xi Xin*), 25g, Radix Rehmanniae (*Sheng Di*), 35g, Radix Ledebouriellae Sesloidis (*Fang Feng*), 25g, Radix Praeparatus

137

Aconiti Carmichaeli (*Zhi Fu Zi*), 30g, Semen Cnidii Monnieri (*She Chuang Zi*), 25g, Radix Angelicae Pubescentis (*Du Huo*), 40g, Radix Achyranthis Bidentatae (*Niu Xi*), 40g, Herba Illicii Lanceolati (*Mang Cao*), 20g, Caulis Et Folium Skimmiae Reevesianae (*Yin Yu*), 25g, blast-fried Rhizoma Zingiberis (*Pao Jiang*), 25g, Herba Dendrobii (*Shi Hu*), 40g

Method of preparation: Place the above 12 medicinals in a large jar after having pestled them into pieces. Soak in 3 *jin* of alcohol and seal the lid. After 7 days, open and remove the dregs.

Method of administration: Take a suitable amount warm before each meal.

Jin Ya Di Fu Jiu (Pyritum & Kochia Wine)

Functions: Relaxes the low back and knees, supplements kidney yang, dispels wind and disinhibits dampness

Mainly treats: Wind stroke insensitivity, difficulty walking and moving about

Ingredients: Pyritum (*Jin Ya Shi*), 20g, Fructus Kochiae Scopariae (*Di Fu Zi*), 30g, prepared Radix Rehmanniae (*Shu Di*), 30g, Caulis Et Folium Sambucudis Javanicae (*Lu Ying Gen*), 30g, Fructus Zanthoxyli Bungeani (*Chuan Jiao*), 120g, Radix Et Rhizoma Notopterygii (*Qiang Huo*), 120g, Radix Praeparatus Aconiti Carmichaeli (*Fu Zi*), 30g, Radix Ledebouriellae Sesloidis (*Fang Feng*), 30g, Herba Cum Radice Asari (*Xi Xin*), 30g, Herba Illicii Lanceolati (*Mang Cao*), 20g

Method of preparation: Pestle the above 10 medicinals into pieces and place in a large jar. Soak in 2 *jin* of white alcohol and seal the lid. Allow to tincture for 3-4 nights in the spring and summer and for

6-7 nights in the fall and winter. Open, remove the dregs, and store for use.

Method of administration: Take 30ml each time. It is normal to feel the alcohol qi, but do not get drunk.

Jin Ya Fu Zi Jiu (Pyritum & Aconite Wine)

Functions: Warms the center and stops pain, quickens the blood and transforms stasis, courses and opens the channels and network vessels, supplements and boosts the liver and kidneys, harmonizes the blood vessels, dispels wind qi, transforms damp turbidity

Mainly treats: Miasmic toxic qi striking humans, mouth and eyes awry, hemiplegia, contracture of the hands and feet, swelling and pain of all the joints, if severe, insensitivity of the small of the low back

Ingredients: Pyritum (*Jin Ya Shi*), 20g, Radix Praeparatus Aconiti Carmichaeli (*Zhi Fu Zi*), 23g, Radix Panacis Ginseng (*Ren Shen*), 18g, Cortex Cinnamomi (*Rou Gui*), 23g, Herba Cistanchis (*Rou Cong Rong*), 15g, Sclerotium Poriae Cocos (*Fu Ling*), 15g, Radix Angelicae Pubescentis (*Du Huo*), 60g, Radix Angelicae Sinensis (*Dang Gui*), 23g, Rhizoma Atractylodis Macrocephalae (*Bai Zhu*), 23g, Fructus Viticis (*Man Jing Zi*), 23g, Radix Ledebouriellae Sesloidis (*Fang Feng*), 23g, Radix Astragali Membranacei (*Huang Qi*), 23g, Fructus Corni Officinalis (*Shan Zhu Yu*), 23g, Herba Cum Radice Asari (*Xi Xin*), 23g, Caulis Et Folium Skimmiae Reevesianae (*Yin Yu*), 20g, Rhizoma Acori Graminei (*Shi Chang Pu*), 23g, Rhizoma Ligustici Wallichii (*Chuan Xiong*), 23g, Cortex Radicis Lycii (*Di Gu Pi*), 23g, Cortex Radicis Acanthopanacis (*Wu Jia Pi*), 23g, Magnetitum (*Ci Shi*), 75g, Radix Salviae Miltiorrhizae (*Dan Shen*), 48g, Cortex Eucommiae Ulmoidis (*Du Zhong*), 52g, Rhizoma Dioscoreae Hypoglaucae (*Bi Xie*), 25g, Radix Achyranthis Bidentatae (*Niu Xi*),

40g, Rhizoma Cibotii Barometsis (*Gou Ji*), 60g, Cortex Magnoliae Officinalis (*Hou Pu*), 23g, Rhizoma Polygonati Odorati (*Yu Zhu*), 15g, Semen Coicis Lachryma-jobi (*Yi Yi Ren*), 120g, Radix Angelicae (*Bai Zhi*), 23g, Tuber Ophiopogonis Japonicae (*Mai Men Dong*), 32g, Herba Dendrobii (*Shi Hu*), 60g, Fructus Citri Seu Ponciri (*Zhi Qiao*), 23g, Radix Platycodi Grandiflori (*Jie Geng*), 23g, Radix Rehmanniae (*Sheng Di*), 250g, Caulis Et Folium Sambucudis Javanicae (*Lu Ying*), 20g, Radix Scutellariae Baicalensis (*Huang Qin*), 23g, Radix Polygalae Tenuifoliae (*Yuan Zhi*), 23g

Method of preparation: Grind the above 37 medicinals into a coarse powder and place in a large cloth bag. Place this bag in a large jar and soak in 5 *jin* of good alcohol. Seal the lid and allow to tincture for 7 days. Then open, remove the dregs, and store for use.

Method of administration: Take 1 teacup warm each day. One may increase the dose to 2-3 teacups. It is normal to feel the alcohol qi. When the condition is better, stop taking.

Jin Ya Ren Shen Jiu (Pyritum & Ginseng Wine)

Functions: Warms the center, stops pain, dispels wind qi, boosts the heart and spleen, relaxes the low back and knees

Mainly treats: Wind toxin foot qi attacking upward the heart and spleen, aphasia

Ingredients: Pyritum (*Jin Ya Shi*), 15g, Herba Cum Radice Asari (*Xi Xin*), 15g, Caulis Et Folium Skimmiae Reevesianae (*Yin Yu*), 15g, Radix Ledebouriellae Sesloidis (*Fang Feng*), 15g, Radix Praeparatus Aconiti Carmichaeli (*Zhi Fu Zi*), 15g, dry Rhizoma Zingiberis (*Gan Jiang*), 15g, Fructus Kochiae Scopariae (*Di Fu Zi*), 15g, Caulis Et Folium Sambucudis Javanicae (*Lu Ying*), 15g, dry Radix Rehmanniae

(*Gan Sheng Di Huang*), 15g, Rhizoma Cimicifugae (*Sheng Ma*), 15g, Radix Panacis Ginseng (*Ren Shen*), 15g, Radix Achyranthis Bidentatae (*Niu Xi*), 23g, Herba Dendrobii (*Shi Hu*), 23g, Radix Angelicae Pubescentis (*Du Huo*), 45g

Method of preparation: Pestle the above 14 medicinals into pieces and place in a large jar. Soak in 2 *jin* of clear alcohol and seal the lid. Allow to tincture for 5 days in the spring and summer and for 7 days in the fall and winter. Open, remove the dregs, and store for use.

Method of administration: Take a suitable amount each time at no fixed schedule. It is normal to feel the power of the alcohol.

Jin Ya Xi Xin Jiu (Pyritum & Asarum Wine)

Functions: Dispels wind dampness, opens the channels and network vessels, disinhibits the joints, strengthens the low back and knees

Mainly treats: Many years wind stroke which has not improved, difficulty to move about, inability to grasp and hold, lockjaw, aphasia, contracture and spasm of the sinews and vessels of the four limbs, wind *bi* wandering about causing aching and pain

Ingredients: Pyritum (*Jin Ya Shi*), 20g, Herba Cum Radice Asari (*Xi Xin*), 30g, Fructus Kochiae Scopariae (*Di Fu Zi*), 30g, dry Rhizoma Zingiberis (*Gan Jiang*), 30g, Radix Et Rhizoma Notopterygii (*Qiang Huo*), 120g, prepared Radix Rehmanniae (*Shu Di*), 30g, Radix Praeparatus Aconiti Carmichaeli (*Zhi Fu Zi*), 30g, Radix Ledebouriel-lae Sesloidis (*Fang Feng*), 30g, Caulis Et Folium Skimmiae Reevesianae (*Yin Yu*), 20g, Fructus Zanthoxyli Bungeani (*Chuan Jiao*), 30g, Caulis Et Folium Sambucudis Javanicae (*Lu Ying Gen*), 20g

Method of preparation: Grind the above 11 medicinals into a fine powder and place in a large jar. Soak in 3 *jin* of clear alcohol and seal the lid. Allow to tincture for 3-4 days in spring and summer and for 6-7 days in fall and winter. Then open, remove the dregs, and store for use.

Method of administration: Take 1 small teacup warm each time. It is common to feel the power of the alcohol. It is also all right to get slightly tipsy.

Yi Ren Bai Lian Jiu (Coix & Ampelopsis Wine)

Functions: Dispels dampness and eliminates *bi*, warms the kidneys and stops pain, opens and disinhibits the sinews and vessels

Mainly treats: Wind, cold, damp qi in the feet, throbbing of the sinews and vessels, *bi* contracture with inability to flex and extend

Ingredients: Stir-fried Semen Coicis Lachryma-jobi (*Yi Yi Ren*), 75g, Radix Ampelopsis (*Bai Lian*), 75g, Radix Albus Paeoniae Lactiflorae (*Bai Shao*), 75g, Semen Zizyphi Spinosae (*Suan Zao Ren*), 75g, dry Rhizoma Zingiberis (*Gan Jiang*), 75g, mix-fried Radix Glycyrrhizae (*Zhi Gan Cao*), 75g, Radix Praeparatus Aconiti Carmichaeli (*Zhi Fu Zi*), 15g

Method of preparation: Pestle the above 7 medicinals into a coarse powder and soak in 3 *jin* of alcohol for 1 night. Then simmer over a low fire. Remove the dregs and decant.

Method of administration: Take 1 small teacup warm before each meal, 3 times per day. Those who do not like to drink alcohol may take as much as they like. It is normal to feel some alcohol qi.

Yi Ren Niu Xi Jiu (Coix & Achyranthes Wine)

Functions: Dispels dampness and eliminates *bi*, disinhibits the joints, boosts the liver and kidneys

Mainly treats: Liver wind sinew and vessel contracture and spasm, inability to flex and extend the joints

Ingredients: Semen Coicis Lachryma-jobi (*Yi Yi Ren*), 120g, Radix Achyranthis Bidentatae (*Niu Xi*), 70g, Radix Rubrus Paeoniae Lactiflorae (*Chi Shao*), 45g, stir-fried Semen Zizyphi Spinosae (*Suan Zao Ren*), 45g, blast-fried dry Rhizoma Zingiberis (*Pao Gan Jiang*), 45g, Radix Praeparatus Aconiti Carmichaeli (*Zhi Fu Zi*), 45g, Semen Biotae Orientalis (*Bai Zi Ren*), 45g, Herba Dendrobii (*Shi Hu*), 45g, mix-fried Radix Glycyrrhizae (*Zhi Gan Cao*), 30g

Method of preparation: Grind the above 9 ingredients into a fine powder and place in a large jar. Soak in 3 *jin* of alcohol. After 7 nights, remove the dregs and store for use.

Method of administration: Take 1-2 small teacups warm at no fixed times.

Contraindications: Pork and fish

Yi Ren Huang Qin Jiu (Coix & Scutellaria Wine)

Functions: Clears heat and resolves toxins, dispels wind dampness

Mainly treats: Foot qi, contracture and spasm of the four limbs, wind toxin aching and pain, neck and upper back contracture (*i.e.*, opisthotonos), a raspy voice

Ingredients: Semen Coicis Lachryma-jobi (*Yi Yi Ren*), 50g, Pulvis Cornu Antelopis (*Ling Yang Jiao Fen*), 10g, Radix Ledebouriellae Sesloidis (*Fang Feng*), 30g, Rhizoma Cimicifugae (*Sheng Ma*), 20g, Radix Gentianae Macrophyllae (*Qin Jiao*), 20g, Radix Scutellariae Baicalensis (*Huang Qin*), 20g, Cortex Radicis Lycii (*Di Gu Pi*), 15g, Fructus Citri Seu Ponciri (*Zhi Qiao*), 15g, Radix Et Rhizoma Notopterygii (*Qiang Huo*), 20g, Radix Achyranthis Bidentatae (*Niu Xi*), 50g, Cortex Radicis Acanthopanacis (*Wu jia Pi*), 30g, Radix Angelicae Pubescentis (*Du Huo*), 20g, slightly stir-fried Fructus Arctii Lappae (*Niu Bang Zi*), 20g, Cortex Cinnamomi (*Rou Gui*), 20g, Semen Cannabis Sativae (*Huo Ma Ren*), 100g, Radix Rehmanniae (*Sheng Di*), 50g

Method of preparation: Pestle the above 16 medicinals into pieces and place in a large jar. Soak in 5 *jin* of alcohol. After 7 days, open and remove the dregs.

Method of administration: Take a suitable amount warm before each meal.

Yi Ren Fang Feng Jiu (Coix & Ledebouriella Wine)

Functions: Boosts the liver and kidneys, eliminates damp *bi*, cures wind tetany

Mainly treats: Kidney viscus wind stroke, low back and knee contracture and spasm, aching and pain

Ingredients: Semen Coicis Lachryma-jobi (*Yi Yi Ren*), 90g, Radix Ledebouriellae Sesloidis (*Fang Feng*), 60g, Radix Achyranthis Bidentatae (*Niu Xi*), 60g, Radix Angelicae Pubescentis (*Du Huo*), 60g, dry Radix Rehmanniae (*Sheng Di Huang*), 60g, stir-fried and parboiled Semen Glycinis Hispidae (*Hei Dou*), 150g, stir-fried Radix

Angelicae Sinensis (*Dang Gui*), 30g, Semen Zizyphi Spinosae (*Suan Zao Ren*), 30g, Rhizoma Ligustici Wallichii (*Chuan Xiong*), 30g, Radix Salviae Miltiorrhizae (*Dan Shen*), 30g, Cortex Cinnamomi (*Rou Gui*), 60g, Radix Praeparatus Aconiti Carmichaeli (*Zhi Fu Zi*), 30g

Method of preparation: Pestle the above 12 medicinals into pieces and place in a large jar. Soak in 4 *jin* of white alcohol and seal the lid. After 5-7 days, open and remove the dregs.

Method of administration: Take 1-2 teacups warm before each meal.

Yin Yu Bi Xie Jiu (Skimmia & Dioscorea Hypoglauca Wine)

Functions: Dispels cold and dampness, strengthens the sinews and bones, stops pain

Mainly treats: Wind, cold, damp *bi*, numbness and insensitivity of the muscles and skin, unbearable aching and pain of the sinews and bones

Ingredients: Caulis Et Folium Skimmiae Reevesianae (*Yin Yu*), 20g, Rhizoma Dioscoreae Hypoglaucae (*Bi Xie*), 30g, Fructus Zanthoxyli Bungeani (*Chuan Jiao*), 30g, Rhizoma Cibotii Barometsis (*Gou Ji*), 30g, Cortex Cinnamomi (*Rou Gui*), 30g, Radix Praeparatus Aconiti Carmichaeli (*Zhi Fu Zi*), 30g, Radix Achyranthis Bidentatae (*Niu Xi*), 30g, Herba Dendrobii (*Shi Hu*), 35g, fresh Rhizoma Zingiberis (*Sheng Jiang*), 35g

Method of preparation: Grind the above 9 medicinals into a fine powder and place in a large jar. Soak in 4 *jin* of alcohol and seal the lid. After 3 nights, open and store for use.

Method of administration: Take 1-2 teacups warm each morning and evening.

Note: After one has drunk half this wine, one may add new alcohol and retincture. When the taste of the medicinals becomes weak, stop.

Chang Song Jiu (Old Pine Wine)

Functions: Dispels wind cold, disinhibits dampness, strengthens the low back and knees

Mainly treats: Wind, cold, damp *bi*, low back pain, weak knees, impotence

Ingredients: Radix Pini (*Song Gen*), 2 *jin* cut up into slices

Method of preparation: Place the slices of Pine Root into a large jar and soak in 2 *jin* of alcohol. Seal the lid. After 7 days, open and remove the dregs.

Method of administration: Take 1-2 teacups warm before each meal.

Fang Feng Song Ye Jiu (Ledebouriella & Pine Needle Wine)

Functions: Dispels wind and eliminates dampness

Mainly treats: Aching and pain of the joints due to invasion of wind dampness, numbness of the four limbs, difficulty moving about

Ingredients: Folium Pini (*Song Ye*), 160g, Herba Ephedrae (*Ma Huang*), 30g, Radix Ledebouriellae Sesloidis (*Fang Feng*), 30g, Radix Praeparatus Aconiti Carmichaeli (*Zhi Fu Zi*), 15g, Radix Angelicae Pubescentis (*Du Huo*), 30g, Radix Gentianae Macrophyllae (*Qin Jiao*), 20g, Cortex Cinnamomi (*Rou Gui*), 20g, Radix Achyranthis Bidentatae (*Niu Xi*), 36g, Radix Rehmanniae (*Sheng Di*), 30g

Method of preparation: Grind the above 9 ingredients into a fine powder and wrap in a cloth bag. Place this in a large jar and soak in 3 *jin* of mellow wine. Seal the lid. After 7 days in spring and fall, 10 days in winter, and 5 days in summer, open and remove the dregs.

Method of administration: Take 1 small teacup (approximately 10ml) warm each time, 3 times per day.

Contraindications: While taking this wine, do not eat foods with toxins, slippery, disinhibiting foods, or foods which stir wind.

Song Jie Di Huang Jiu (Pine Node & Rehmannia Wine)

Functions: Dispels wind, disinhibits dampness, warms the center

Mainly treats: Foot qi with contracture of the sinews, pulling pain of the four limbs, possible weakness of the feet, inhibited joints

Ingredients: Nodus Pini (*Song Jie*), 100g, Radix Rehmanniae (*Sheng Di*), 50g, Cortex Cinnamomi (*Rou Gui*), 20g, Radix Gentianae Macrophyllae (*Qin Jiao*), 50g, Radix Ledebouriellae Sesloidis (*Fang Feng*), 20g, Fructus Arctii Lappae (*Niu Bang Zi*), 100g, Radix Salviae Miltiorrhizae (*Dan Shen*), 30g, Rhizoma Dioscoreae Hypoglaucae (*Bi Xie*), 30g, Fructus Xanthii (*Cang Er Zi*), 30g, Radix Angelicae Pubescentis (*Du Huo*), 30g, stir-fried till fragrant Semen Cannabis

Sativae (*Huo Ma Ren*), 100g, Radix Achyranthis Bidentatae (*Niu Xi*), 50g

Method of preparation: Grind the above 12 medicinals into a fine powder and place them in a large jar. Soak in 4 *jin* of alcohol. After 7 days, open and drink.

Method of administration: Take a suitable amount warm before each meal.

Sheng Di Jia Pi Jiu (Raw Rehmannia & Acanthopanax Wine)

Functions: Dispels wind dampness, clears heat, stops pain, soothes the sinews

Mainly treats: Vexatious heat, aching and pain, contracture and spasm of the sinews and vessels, inhibition of the joints, difficulty moving about

Ingredients: Cortex Radicis Acanthopanacis (*Wu Jia Pi*), 30g, Semen Coicis Lachryma-jobi (*Yi Yi Ren*), 50g, Pulvis Cornu Antelopis (*Ling Yang Jiao Fen*), 20g, Radix Ledebouriellae Sesloidis (*Fang Feng*), 30g, Radix Rehmanniae (*Sheng Di*), 60g, Radix Angelicae Pubescentis (*Du Huo*), 30g, Radix Arctii Lappae (*Niu Bang Gen, i.e.,* Burdock Root), 60g, Cortex Cinnamomi (*Rou Gui*), 10g, Radix Achyranthis Bidentatae (*Niu Xi*), 50g, stir-fried and parboiled Semen Glycinis Hispidae (*Hei Dou*), 60g, Cortex Erythriniae (*Hai Tong Pi*), 20g, Semen Cannabis Sativae (*Huo Ma Ren*), 60g

Method of preparation: Grind the above 12 ingredients into a fine powder and place in a large jar. Soak in 4 *jin* of mellow wine and seal the lid. After 7 nights, open and drink.

Method of administration: Take a suitable amount on an empty stomach before each meal.

Yin Yu Yi Ren Jiu (Skimmia & Coix Wine)

Functions: Scatters cold, dispels wind, and eliminates dampness

Mainly treats: Contracture and spasm of the sinews and vessels, inability to extend

Ingredients: Caulis et Folium Skimmiae Reevesianae (*Yin Yu*), 20g, Rhizoma Bletillae Striatae (*Bai Ji*), 30g, Semen Coicis Lachryma-jobi (*Yi Yi Ren*), 30g, Radix Rubrus Paeoniae Lactiflorae (*Chi Shao*), 30g, Cortex Cinnamomi (*Rou Gui*), 30g, Radix Achyranthis Bidentatae (*Niu Xi*), 30g, stir-fried Semen Zizyphi Spinosae (*Suan Zao Ren*), 30g, blast-fried Rhizoma Zingiberis (*Pao Jiang*), 15g, Radix Praeparatus Aconiti Carmichaeli (*Zhi Fu Zi*), 30g, mix-fried Radix Glycyrrhizae (*Zhi Gan Cao*), 15g

Method of preparation: Grind the above 10 medicinals into a fine powder and wrap them in a cloth bag. Place in a large jar and soak in 2 *jin* of alcohol. Seal the lid. After 7 nights, open the lid and remove the dregs. Store for use.

Method of administration: Take a suitable amount warm at no fixed times.

Jiu Wei Yi Ren Jiu (Nine Flavors Coix Wine)

Functions: Dispels wind and disinhibits dampness

Mainly treats: Foot *bi* pain

Ingredients: Semen Coicis Lachryma-jobi (*Yi Yi Ren*), 60g, Radix Achyranthis Bidentatae (*Niu Xi*), 60g, Cortex Erythriniae (*Hai Tong Pi*), 30g, Cortex Radicis Acanthopanacis (*Wu Jia Pi*), 30g, Radix Angelicae Pubescentis (*Du Huo*), 30g, Radix Ledebouriellae Sesloidis (*Fang Feng*), 30g, Cortex Eucommiae Ulmoidis (*Du Zhong*), 30g, prepared Radix Rehmanniae (*Shu Di*), 45g, Rhizoma Atractylodis Macrocephalae (*Bai Zhu*), 20g

Method of preparation: Grind the above 9 ingredients into a fine powder and wrap them in a cloth bag. Place in a large jar and soak in 4 *jin* of alcohol. Allow to tincture for 3 days in the spring and summer and for 7 days in the fall and winter. Then open the lid, remove the dregs, and store for use.

Method of administration: Take 15-20ml warm and before meals each time, 3 times per day.

Shou Wu Yi Ren Jiu (Polygonum Multiflorum & Coix Wine)

Functions: Nourishes the blood, dispels wind dampness, stops pain

Mainly treats: Blood vacuity wind dampness low back pain, numbness of the four extremities, dizziness and vertigo

Ingredients: Processed Radix Polygoni Multiflori (*Zhi Shou Wu*), 180g, Semen Coicis Lachryma-jobi (*Yi Yi Ren*), 120g

Method of preparation: Soak the above 2 ingredients in 1kg of white alcohol for 15 days.

Method of administration: Take 2 small teacups each time, 2 times per day.

Tian Ma Jiu (Gastrodia Wine)

Functions: Extinguishes wind and settles tetany

Mainly treats: Numbness of the body and limbs, inability to flex and extend the hands and feet

Ingredients: Rhizoma Gastrodiae Elatae (*Tian Ma*), 24g, Radix Achyranthis Bidentatae (*Niu Xi*), 24g, stir-fried Cortex Eucommiae Ulmoidis (*Du Zhong*), 24g

Method of preparation: Cut the above ingredients into pieces and soak in 1kg of yellow (*i.e.*, rice) wine for 7 days.

Method of administration: Take 1 teacup each time, 2 times per day.

7

Heat-clearing, Dampness-disinhibiting Wines

Although alcohol consumption is a leading cause of damp heat evils, damp heat, liver heat, and toxic heat conditions can, according to Li Shi-zhen's *Ben Cao Gang Mu (Complete Outline of the Materia Medica)*, also be treated by alcoholic tinctures. However, this method of treatment is mostly appropriate for the elderly who have a combination of dampness and heat with underlying vacuity and insufficiency. I do not recommend this method of administration in young or middle-aged patients. As the reader will see, there are only a few formulas in this section as compared to other sections in this book. This underscores the fact that alcohol is typically contraindicated in damp heat conditions.

Ju Hua Jiu (Chrysanthemum Wine)

Functions: Clears heat and dispels wind, brightens the eyes and resolves toxins

Mainly treats: Dizziness and vertigo, red, swollen, painful eyes, painful, swollen clove sores

Ingredients: Flos Chrysanthemi Morifolii (*Ju Hua*), 250g, raw Radix Rehmanniae (*Sheng Di*), 15g, Radix Angelicae Sinensis (*Dang Gui*), 15g, Fructus Lycii Chinensis (*Gou Qi Zi*), 30g

Method of preparation: Soak the above medicinals in 2 *jin* of white alcohol and seal the lid. After 5 days, open the lid, remove the dregs, and decant.

Method of administration: Take 15-30ml slowly, slowly each time at no fixed schedule.

Jin Hua Jiu (Golden Flower Wine)

Functions: Clears heat and disinhibits dampness

Mainly treats: Oral sores and bleeding gums

Ingredients: Cortex Phellodendri (*Huang Bai*), 90g, Rhizoma Coptidis Chinensis (*Huang Lian*), 15g, Fructus Gardeniae Jasminoidis (*Zhi Zi*), 30g

Method of preparation: Place the above 3 ingredients in a large jar and soak in 500ml of red rice wine. Then place this jar in a large pan of water and bring to a a boil 100 times. Allow to cool and then remove the dregs. Store for use.

Method administration: Take 20ml on an empty stomach at no fixed schedule. When cured, stop.

Dan Shen Jiu (Salvia Wine)

Functions: Percolates dampness and disinhibits water, disperses stasis and resolves binding, dispels wind

Mainly treats: Upper abdominal water drum distention, swelling and fullness of the foot and lower leg, distressed rapid breathing due to eating

Ingredients: Radix Salviae Miltiorrhizae (*Dan Shen*), 27g, Lignum Buchnerae Cruciata (*Gui Yu Jian*), 27g, Radix Gentianae Macrophyllae (*Qin Jiao*), 18g, Rhizoma Anemarrhenae (*Zhi Mu*), 18g, Sclerotium Polypori Umbellati (*Zhu Ling*), 27g, Rhizoma Atractylodis Macrocephalae (*Bai Zhu*), 27g, Herba Sargassii (*Hai Zao*), 10g, Sclerotium Rubrum Poriae Cocos (*Chi Fu Ling*), 18g, Cortex Cinnamomi (*Rou Gui*), Radix Angelicae Pubescentis (*Du Huo*), 15g

Method of preparation: Place the above 10 medicinals in a large jar and soak in 2 *jin* of alcohol. Seal the lid and allow to tincture for 5 days. Then open the lid, remove the dregs, and store for use.

Method of administration: Take 20ml each time 3 times per day.

Contraindications: Do not take this formula if there is spleen vacuity diarrhea. Nor should pregnant women use this prescription.

Niu Bang Song Jie Jiu (Burdock Root & Pine Node Wine)

Functions: Clears heat and disinhibits dampness

Mainly treats: Heart spirit vexation and oppression, lower leg and foot swelling and fullness, a heavy body, and lack of strength

Ingredients: Nodus Pini (*Fei Song Jie*), 120g, raw Radix Rehmanniae (*Sheng Di*), 30g, Cortex Cinnamomi (*Rou Gui*), 10g, Radix Salviae Miltiorrhizae (*Dan Shen*), 30g, Rhizoma Dioscoreae Hypoglaucae (*Bi Xie*), 20g, Semen Cannabis Sativae (*Huo Ma Ren*), 120g,

155

Radix Achyranthis Bidentatae (*Niu Xi*), 30g, raw Radix Arctii Lappae (*Sheng Niu Bang Gen, i.e.*, Burdock Root), 30g

Method of preparation: Grind the above 8 medicinals into a fine powder and place in a large jar. Soak in 3 *jin* of alcohol and seal the lid. After 5 days, open, remove the dregs, and store for use.

Method of administration: Take 1 teacup warm before each meal.

Yi Yi Ren Jiu (Coix Wine)

Functions: Fortifies the spleen, disinhibits water and percolates dampness, clears heat

Mainly treats: Abdominal distention, diarrhea, edema, inhibited urination, foot qi and swollen foot, *bi* pain of the four extremities, difficulty bending and flexing, numbness and insensitivity of the muscles and skin, lung abscess, coughing and vomiting pussy phlegm

Ingredients: Semen Coicis Lachryma-jobi (*Yi Yi Ren*), 250g

Method of preparation: Place the above ingredient in a large jar and soak in 2 *jin* of alcohol. Place this jar in a large pan of water and boil. Allow to cool, remove the dregs, and store for use.

Method of administration: Take 2-3 teacups 3 times per day.

Cang Zhu Chi Jiu (Atractylodes & Fermented Soybean Wine)

Functions: Diffuses obstruction and dispels dampness, clears and eliminates vexatious heat

Mainly treats: Wind toxin weak lower legs, numbness and lack of strength, foot and lower leg swelling and distention, vomiting, inability to eat, abdominal pain, dysentery, headache, fever

Ingredients: Semen Praeparatum Sojae (*Dan Dou Chi*), 1 *jin*, Rhizoma Atractylodis (*Cang Zhu*), 50g

Method of preparation: Place the prepared soybeans in a large jar and soak in 2 *jin* of clear alcohol. After 3 nights, add the powdered Atractylodes. After another 4 days, open, remove the dregs, and store for use.

Method of administration: Slowly, slowly drink whatever amount one wishes at no fixed schedule.

San Ren Jiu (Three Seeds Wine)

Functions: Diffuses, transforms, and smoothes away swelling, clears heat and disinhibits dampness

Mainly treats: The initial stages of dampness and warmth, summer-heat heat and dampness, headache, a heavy body, chest oppression, devitalized appetite

Ingredients: Semen Pruni Armeniacae (*Xing Ren*), 50g, Talcum (*Hua Shi*), 50g, Medulla Tetrapanacis Papyriferi (*Tong Cao*), 30g, Folium Lophatheri Gracilis (*Dan Zhu Ye*), 30g, Cortex Magnoliae Officinalis (*Hou Po*), 30g, raw Semen Coicis Lachryma-jobi (*Sheng Yi Yi Ren*), 50g, Rhizoma Pinelliae Ternatae (*Ban Xia*), 30g, Fructus Cardamomi (*Bai Dou Kou Ren*), 20g

157

Method of preparation: Grind the above 8 medicinals into a fine powder and place in a large jar. Soak in 3 *jin* of red rice wine After 7 nights, open, remove the dregs, and decant.

Method of administration: Take 20ml each time 3 times per day.

Contraindications: Avoid exposure to wind while taking this prescription. This formula should not be used by pregnant women.

Qing Hao Jiu (Artemisia Apiacea Wine)

Functions: Clears heat and cools the blood, resolves summerheat, recedes vacuity heat

Mainly treats: Steaming bones and tidal fever, no sweating, evenings feverish, mornings cool, epistaxis, summertime common cold, malarial disease, alternating hot and cold, chest glomus, nausea and vomiting, jaundice, inhibited urination

Ingredients: Herba Artemisiae Apiaceae (*Qing Hao*), 300g

Method of preparation: Grind the above medicinal into a fine powder and place in a large jar. Soak in 2 *jin* of alcohol and seal the lid. After 7 days, remove the dregs and store for use.

Method of administration: Take as much as one wishes at no fixed schedule.

Tong Cao Gen (Tetrapanax Papyriferus Wine)

Functions: Disinhibits water and percolates dampness, clears heat and opens the channels

Mainly treats: Edema, strangury diseases (*i.e.*, benign prostatic hypertrophy and chronic prostatitis), vexatious heat in the chest disquieting the heart, scanty, frequent urination, breast milk not free-flowing

Ingredients: Medulla Tetrapanacis Papyriferi (*Tong Cao*), 250g, Medulla Junci Effusi (*Deng Xin Cao*), 30g

Method of preparation: Grind the above 2 ingredients into a fine powder and place in a large jar. Soak in 2 *jin* of alcohol and seal the lid. After 7 days, open and remove the dregs.

Method of administration: Take as much as one wants, slowly, slowly at no fixed schedule.

Contraindications: Pregnant women should not use this prescription. It is also not appropriate to use this formula in cases of qi vacuity without damp heat.

8

Fortifying the Spleen & Harmonizing the Stomach Wines

The wines in this chapter fortify the spleen and harmonize the stomach. That means that they treat nausea, vomiting, lack of appetite, loose stools, abdominal pain, abdominal distention, and indigestion. According to the *Nei Jing (Inner Classic)*, the *yang ming* begins to decline at around 35 years of age. The *yang ming* here refers to the power of digestion. As one ages, one commonly finds that they can "stomach" less and less foods. The wines in this chapter are designed to off-set this aspect of aging and to treat the most common complaints associated with indigestion.

Qing Mei Jiu (Green Plum Wine)

Functions: Engenders fluids, revitalizes the appetite, promotes digestion, kills worms (*i.e.*, parasites)

Mainly treats: Devitalized appetite, poor digestion, round worm abdominal pain

Ingredients: Fructus Immaturus Pruni (*Qing Mei*), 30g

Method of preparation: Place the Green Plums in a jar and soak in 100ml of yellow (*i.e.*, rice) wine. Then place this jar in a pan of water and bring to a boil. Cook for 20 minutes. Remove the dregs.

Method of administration: Take 20ml warm as needed.

Ban Xia Ren Shen Jiu (Pinellia & Ginseng Wine)

Functions: Harmonizes the stomach and downbears counterflow, opens binding and scatters glomus

Mainly treats: Stomach qi disharmony, mutual binding of cold and heat, glomus and hardness below the heart, nausea and upward counterflow (*i.e.*, tendency to vomiting), borborygmus and downward disinhibition (*i.e.*, tendency to diarrhea), lack of desire for food and drink, bodily fatigue and lack of strength

Ingredients: Rhizoma Pinelliae Ternatae (*Ban Xia*), 30g, Radix Scutellariae Baicalensis (*Huang Qin*), 30g, dry Rhizoma Zingiberis (*Gan Jiang*), 20g, Radix Panacis Ginseng (*Ren Shen*), 20g, mix-fried Radix Glycyrrhizae (*Zhi Gan Cao*), 20g, Rhizoma Coptidis Chinensis (*Huang Lian*), 6g, Fructus Zizyphi Jujubae (*Da Zao*), 10g

Method of preparation: Pestle the above 7 ingredients and place in a large jar. Soak in 1.5 *jin* of alcohol. After 5 days add 1 *jin* of cold water and stir. Remove the dregs and store for use.

Method of administration: Take 20ml 1 time each morning and night.

Yi Pi Jiu (Boost the Spleen Wine)

Functions: Boosts the middle and opens the bowels

Mainly treats: Chilly pain in the abdomen, constipation or prolonged dysentery

Ingredients: Dry Rhizoma Zingiberis (*Gan Jiang*), 30g, Radix Glycyrrhizae (*Gan Cao*), 30g, Radix Et Rhizoma Rhei (*Da Huang*),

30g, Radix Panacis Ginseng (*Ren Shen*), 20g, Radix Praeparatus Aconiti Carmichaeli (*Zhi Fu Zi*), 20g

Method of preparation: Grind the above 5 medicinals into a fine powder and place in a large jar. Soak in 1 *jin* of yellow wine (*i.e.*, rice wine). After 5 days, open the lid and remove the dregs. Then store for use.

Method of administration: Take 10-20ml warm 1 time each morning and night.

Jiang Fu Jiu (Ginger & Aconite Wine)

Functions: Warms the middle and scatters cold, rescues yang and opens the vessels, warms the lungs and transforms rheum

Mainly treats: Chilly pain of the heart and abdomen, nausea and vomiting, diarrhea, indigestion, cold rheum wheezing and coughing, white phlegm or clear, watery phlegm, chilled limbs, sweating

Ingredients: Dry Rhizoma Zingiberis (*Gan Jiang*), 60g, Radix Praeparatus Aconiti Carmichaeli (*Zhi Fu Zi*), 40g

Method of preparation: Grind the above 2 medicinals into a fine powder and place in a large jar. Soak in 1 *jin* of yellow (*i.e.*, rice) wine and seal the lid. After 7 nights, open the lid and use.

Method of administration: Take 1-2 teacups 3 times per day warm and before meals.

Contraindications: This formula is not appropriate if there is yin vacuity internal heat or fire heat abdominal pain.

Fu Zi Jiu (Aconite Wine)

Functions: Warms the middle and scatters cold, stops pain

Mainly treats: Lack of warmth of the four limbs, dribbling and dripping of chilly sweat, a greyish white facial color, vomiting, chilly diarrhea, fear of cold, chilly pain within the abdomen, aching joints

Ingredients: Radix Praeparatus Aconiti Carmichaeli (*Zhi Fu Zi*), 30g

Method of preparation: Grind the above ingredient in a mortar until it is broken up to the size of large beans. Then place in a large jar and soak in 1 *jin* of mellow wine for from 3-5 days. Then open and use.

Method of administration: Take 1 small teacup each time. If one experiences a slight numbness, one is taking too much.

Ling Zhu Jiu (Poria & Atractylodes Wine)

Functions: Supplements the spleen and dries dampness, harmonizes the center and dispels phlegm

Mainly treats: Diminished appetite, abdominal distention, indigestion, diarrhea, phlegm rheum coughing, edema, inhibited urination

Ingredients: Rhizoma Atractylodis Macrocephalae (*Bai Zhu*), 1 *jin*, Sclerotium Poriae Cocos (*Fu Ling*), 1/2 *jin*

Method of preparation: Soak these 2 ingredients in 5 *jin* of yellow wine (*i.e.*, rice wine) for 10 days. Then remove the dregs and store for use.

Method of administration: Take 1-2 teacups 3 times per day on an empty stomach.

Suo Sha Jiu (Amomum Wine)

Functions: Moves the qi and harmonizes the middle, opens the stomach and disperses food

Mainly treats: Distention and fullness of the chest and abdomen, devitalized appetite, indigestion, *shan* qi, vomiting, stomach pain, diarrhea, dysentery

Ingredients: Fructus Amomi (*Suo Sha Ren*), 60g

Method of preparation: Grind into powder the above medicinal and place in a large jar. Soak in 1 *jin* of yellow wine (*i.e.*, rice wine). After 3-5 days, open and use.

Method of administration: Take 15-20ml 3 times per day warm and after meals.

Contraindications: This formula is not appropriate in case of yin vacuity or replete heat.

Hui Xiang Jiu (Fennel Wine)

Functions: Scatters cold and stops pain, opens the stomach and leads away food

Mainly treats: Cold *shan* lower abdominal pain, testicular pain affecting the lower abdomen, women's abnormal vaginal discharge,

165

epigastric pain, distention, and oppression, no desire for food or drink, vomiting

Ingredients: Stir-fried Fructus Foeniculi Vulgaris (*Xiao Hui Xiang*), 120g

Method of preparation: Place the above ingredient in a large jar and soak in 1 *jin* of yellow wine (*i.e.*, rice wine). Place this jar in a pan of water and bring to a boil several times. Then remove and allow to cool, open, and use.

Method of administration: Take 1-2 teacups 3 times per day warm and before meals.

Zhu Ling Ren Dong Jiu (Atractylodes, Poria & Caulis Lonicerae Wine)

Functions: Supplements the spleen and harmonizes the stomach, boosts the wisdom and quiets the spirit, brightens the eyes and improves hearing, dispels wind and dampness

Mainly treats: Spleen vacuity accumulation of dampness, epigastric glomus and fullness, heart palpitations, dizziness, heaviness of the low back and legs

Ingredients: Rhizoma Atractylodis Macrocephalae (*Bai Zhu*), 60g, Sclerotium Poriae Cocos (*Fu Ling*), 60g, Flos Chrysanthemi Morifolii (*Gan Ju Hua*), 60g, Caulis Lonicerae Japonicae (*Ren Dong Teng*), 40g

Method of preparation: First finely chop the Atractylodes, Poria, and Caulis Lonicerae. Then place these and the sweet Chrysanthemum in a large jar. Soak in 3 *jin* of mellow wine and seal the lid. After 7

days, open and add 2 *jin* of cold water. Remove the dregs and store for use.

Method of administration: Take 1-2 medium teacups 1-2 times per day warm and on an empty stomach.

Shan Zha Jiu (Hawthorne Berry Wine)

Functions: Promotes digestion and disperses stagnant food

Mainly treats: Accumulation and stagnation of meat, epigastric and abdominal distention and oppression

Ingredients: Fructus Crataegi (*Shan Zha*), 250g, Cortex Cinnamomi (*Rou Gui*), 250g, Fructus Ziziphi Jujubae (*Da Zao*), 30g, Brown Sugar (*Hong Tang*), 30g

Method of preparation: Grind the above ingredients into pieces and place in a large jar. Soak in 1kg of rice wine for 10 days. Remove the dregs and store for use.

Method of administration: Take one small teacup each time, two times per day.

Shen Qu Jiu (Medicated Leaven Wine)

Functions: Promotes digestion and disperses stagnant food

Mainly treats: Food stagnation, indigestion

Ingredients: Massa Medica Fermentata (*Shen Qu*), 90g

Method of preparation: Grind the above medicinal into pieces and place in a large jar. Soak in 1kg of rice wine for 7 days.

Method of administration: Take 30ml each time, 2 times per day.

9

Wines for Women's Diseases

Medicinal wines used in TCM gynecology primarily treat acute conditions where speedy remedy is important. These include threatened abortion, dysmenorrhea, and profuse uterine bleeding. Medicinal wines are also used in the treatment of postpartum wind stroke. In general, Chinese medical theory holds that women tend to be vacuous and even cold postpartum. Therefore, the warming and nourishing properties of alcohol are appropriate. In addition, in cases of postpartum wind stroke (*i.e.*, postpartum convulsive disorders), the woman may not be lucid and in full control of either her faculties or bodily functions. Therefore, it is important to get into the woman relatively concentrated and powerful medicine as quickly as possible but without much swallowing. In such cases, drinking large cupfuls of decoctions or trying to swallow pills tend to be difficult. And finally, medicinal wines are also used to treat both insufficient lactation and mastitis. This is most likely due to alcohol's tropism for the liver channel and the fact that an internal branch of the liver channel travels to the breast.

Hong Lan Hua Jiu (Carthamus Wine)

Function: Quickens the blood and transforms stasis

Mainly treats: Women's abdominal piercing pain due to blood stasis accompanying a variety of women's diseases

Ingredients: Flos Carthami Tinctorii (*Hong Hua*), 30g

Method of preparation: Place the Carthamus in 200ml of alcohol and decoct until reduced by half.

Method of administration: Take 50ml warm as needed. If the pain does not cease, take the other 50ml.

Dang Gui Jiu (Dang Gui Wine)

Functions: Quickens the blood and transforms stasis

Mainly treats: Menstrual irregularity, dysmenorrhea, incomplete miscarriage, infertility

Ingredients: Radix Angelicae Sinensis (*Dang Gui*), 20g, Flos Carthami Tinctorii (*Hong Hua*), 10g

Method of preparation: Soak in 50ml of white alcohol for 48 hours. Then add 100ml of white alcohol more. Remove the dregs.

Method of administration: Each time take 30ml, 3 times per day.

Gua Lou Jiu (Trichosanthis Wine)

Functions: Opens the breasts (*i.e.*, promotes the flow of breast milk)

Mainly treats: Agalactia

Ingredients: Fructus Trichosanthis Kirlowii (*Gua Lou*), 1 piece

Method of preparation: Pestle 1 ripe fruit into a pulpy mash and then boil in 5 teacups of wine till 2 teacups of liquid remain. Remove the dregs and store for use.

Method administration: Take 1 teacup warm each time at no fixed schedule.

Tong Cao Jiu (Tetrapanax Papyriferus Wine)

Functions: Opens the breasts

Mainly treats: Agalactia

Ingredients: Medulla Tetrapanacis Papyriferi (*Tong Cao*), 30g, powdered Stalactitum (*Shi Zhong Ru*), 60g

Method of preparation: Place the above 2 ingredients in a large jar, soak in 400ml of rice wine, and seal the lid. Place next to a fire and allow to simmer slowly. After 3 nights, open and use.

Method of administration: Drink slowly, at no fixed schedule.

Yong Quan Jiu (Gushing Spring Wine)

Functions: Harmonizes the blood and opens the channels

Mainly treats: Postpartum breast milk not flowing freely

Ingredients: Semen Vaccariae Segetalis (*Wang Bu Liu Xing*), 10g, Radix Trichosanthis Kirlowii (*Tian Hua Fen*), 10g, Radix Angelicae Sinensis (*Dang Gui*), 7g, stir-fried Squama Manitis Pentadactylae (*Chuan Shan Jia*), 5g, Radix Glycyrrhizae (*Gan Cao*), 10g

Method of preparation: Grind the above 5 ingredients into a fine powder.

Method of administration: Take 7g of the above powder and boil in 2 teacups of yellow wine (*i.e.*, rice wine) down to 1 teacup. Take warm 2 times per day.

Pu Gong Ying Jiu (Dandelion Wine)

Functions: Resolves toxins

Mainly treats: Breast abscesses, breast distention and pain

Ingredients: Fresh Herba Cum Radice Taraxaci Mongolici (*Xian Pu Gong Ying*), 1 handful

Method of preparation: Place the Dandelion in a mortar and smash with a pestle, mixing the resulting mash with 1 small teacup of alcohol. Remove the dregs and use.

Method of administration: Drink warm at no fixed schedule any amount one wants.

Di Yu Chang Pu Jiu (Sanguisorba & Acorus Wine)

Functions: Stops bleeding

Mainly treats: Postpartum uterine bleeding

Ingredients: Rhizoma Acori Graminei (*Shi Chang Pu*), 20g, Radix Sanguisorbae (*Di Yu*), 50g, Radix Angelicae Sinensis (*Dang Gui*), 40g

Method of preparation: Grind the above 3 medicinals into a fine powder and place in a large jar. Soak in 500ml of yellow wine (*i.e.*, rice wine) and boil until 1 teacup remains. Remove the dregs and use.

Method administration: Divide into 3 doses and take warm before meals.

Ji Gen Jiu (Cirsius & Cephalanoplos Wine)

Functions: Stops bleeding

Mainly treats: Women's uterine bleeding which will not stop due to heat

Ingredients: Herba Cirsii Japonici Et Cephalanoploris Segeti (*Da Xiao Ji*), 200g @

Method of preparation: Place the 2 above medicinals in a large jar and soak in 600ml of alcohol. After 5 days, open the lid, remove the dregs, and store for use.

Method of administration: Drink at will.

Jiao Ai Jiu (Donkey Skin Glue & Mugwort Wine)

Functions: Quiets the fetus

Mainly treats: Threatened miscarriage, restless fetus

Ingredients: Gelatinum Corii Asini (*E Jiao*), 30g, Folium Artemisiae Argyii (*Ai Ye*), 20g, Rhizoma Ligustici Wallichii (*Chuan Xiong*), 20g, Radix Paeoniae Lactiflorae (*Shao Yao*), 20g, Radix Glycyrrhizae (*Gan Cao*), 20g, Radix Angelicae Sinensis (*Dang Gui*), 30g, raw Radix Rehmanniae (*Sheng Di*), 30g

Method of preparation: Decoct the above ingredients in 1/2 *jin* each of water and yellow wine (*i.e.*, rice wine) until reduced to 1/2 *jin*. Remove the dregs and divide into 3 portions.

Method of administration: Take 1 portion each morning, noon, and night.

Bai Zhu Jiu (Atractylodes Wine)

Functions: Quiets the fetus

Mainly treats: Spleen qi vacuity weakness during pregnancy, restless fetus (*i.e.*, threatened abortion)

Ingredients: Rhizoma Atractylodis Macrocephalae (*Bai Zhu*), 60g

Method of preparation: Grind the above medicinal into a fine powder and store for use.

Method of administration: For each dose, bring to a boil 6gm of the above medicinal in 50ml of yellow wine (*i.e.*, rice wine) several times. Then drink warm. Take 1 time each morning, noon, and night.

Can Sha Dou Lin Jiu (Silkworm & Black Soybean Filtered Wine)

Functions: Dispels wind

Mainly treats: All sorts of postpartum wind stroke diseases

Ingredients: Semen Glycinis Hispidae (*Hei Dou*), 1/2 *jin*, Bombyx Batryticatus (*Can Sha*), 250g

174

Method of preparation: Stir-fry the Black Soybeans in 2 *jin* of alcohol and then remove the dregs. Then place the resulting liquid in a large jar and add the Silkworms. Allow to tincture for 5 days, remove those dregs, and decant.

Method of administration: Take 50ml warm 2 times during the day and 1 time at night.

Huang Qi Fang Feng Jiu (Astragalus & Ledebouriella Wine)

Functions: Eliminates wind and stops pain, quickens the blood and opens the channels

Mainly treats: Postpartum wind stroke, hemiplegia, inhibited speech, lower back and lower extremity aching and pain, lack of strength

Ingredients: Radix Astragali Membranacei (*Huang Qi*), 60g, Fructus Zanthoxyli Bungeani (*Shu Jiao*), 60g, Rhizoma Atractylodis Macrocephalae (*Bai Zhu*), 60g, Radix Achyranthis Bidentatae (*Niu Xi*), 60g, Radix Puerariae Lobatae (*Ge Gen*), 60g, Radix Ledebouriellae Sesloidis (*Fang Feng*), 90g, mix-fried Radix Glycyrrhizae (*Zhi Gan Cao*), 30g, Fructus Corni Officinalis (*Shan Zhu Yu*), 30g, Radix Praeparatus Aconiti Carmichaeli (*Zhi Fu Zi*), 30g, Radix Gentianae Macrophyllae (*Qin Jiao*), 30g, blast-fried Rhizoma Zingiberis (*Pao Jiang*), 30g, Radix Angelicae Sinensis (*Dang Gui*), 30g, processed Radix Aconiti (*Zhi Wu Tou*), 30g, Radix Panacis Ginseng (*Ren Shen*), 30g, Radix Angelicae Pubescentis (*Du Huo*), 10g, Cortex Cinnamomi (*Rou Gui*), 3g

Method of preparation: Grind the above 16 medicinals into a fine powder and place in a large jar. Soak in 3 *jin* of alcohol and seal the lid. Allow to tincture for 3 days in the spring and summer and for 5

175

days in the fall and winter. Then open the lid, remove the dregs, and store for use.

Method of administration: Take 1 teacup warm at no fixed schedule.

Qiang Huo Jiu (Notopterygium Wine)

Functions: Resolves tetany and stops pain

Mainly treats: Postpartum wind stroke abdominal pain

Ingredients: Radix Et Rhizoma Notopterygii (*Qiang Huo*), 15g

Method of preparation: Boil the above single ingredient in 1 teacup of alcohol down to 1/2 teacup or approximately 35ml.

Method of administration: Take warm as needed.

Du Huo Ren Shen Jiu (Angelica Pubescens & Ginseng Wine)

Functions: Dispels wind and resolves tetany, supplements vacuity and clears heat

Mainly treats: Postpartum wind stroke, fatigue, excessive sweating, fever, headache

Ingredients: Radix Angelicae Pubescentis (*Du Huo*), 45g, Cortex Dictamni Dasycarpae (*Bai Xian Pi*), 15g, Radix Et Rhizoma Notopterygii (*Qiang Huo*), 30g, Radix Panacis Ginseng (*Ren Shen*), 20g

176

Method of preparation: Grind the above 4 medicinals into a fine powder.

Method of administration: Take 10g of this medicinal powder and add to 7 parts water and 3 parts alcohol. Boil down to 7/10 and remove the dregs. Take warm as needed.

Ji Sheng Hei Dou Jiu (Loranthus & Black Soybean Wine)

Functions: Resolves tetany and stops pain

Mainly treats: Postpartum wind stroke, lower and upper back aching and pain, lockjaw

Ingredients: Semen Glycinis Hispidae (*Hei Dou*), 250g, Ramus Loranthis Seu Visci (*Sang Ji Sheng*), 200g

Method of preparation: Grind the Loranthus into a fine powder and place in a large jar. Soak in 3 *jin* of alcohol. Next, stir-fry the Black Soybeans till fragrant and also put in the alcohol. After 5 days, remove the dregs and store for use.

Method of administration: Take 1 small teacup warm as needed.

Zhong Yu Jiu (Jade Wine)

Functions: Quickens the blood and opens the channels (or menses), regulates and rectifies the qi and blood

Mainly treats: Women's menstrual irregularity, female infertility, qi and blood insufficiency

177

Ingredients: Radix Angelicae Sinensis (*Dang Gui*), 150g, Radix Polygalae Tenuifoliae (*Yuan Zhi*), 150g

Method of preparation: Place these two ingredients in a large jar, soak in 3 *jin* of sweet wine (*i.e.*, brandy or sherry), and seal the lid. After 7 days, open the lid, remove the dregs, and store for use.

Method of administration: Take as much as one wants warm in the evening, but do not get drunk.

Xiang Fu Gen Jiu (Cyperus Wine)

Functions: Rectifies the qi and resolves depression, regulates the menses and stops pain

Mainly treats: Chest and lateral costal distention and pain, epigastric aching and pain, devitalized appetite, irregular menstruation, breast distention and pain, depression and oppression affecting the heart

Ingredients: Rhizoma Cyperi Rotundi (*Xiang Fu*), 60g

Method of preparation: Cut the Cyperus into slices and place in a large jar. Soak in 1/2 *jin* each of water and white alcohol. Allow to tincture for 5 days. Remove the dregs and store for use.

Method of administration: Drink repeatedly at no fixed schedule.

Shao Yao Huang Qi Jiu (Peony & Astragalus Wine)

Functions: Regulates the menses and stops abnormal vaginal discharge

Mainly treats: Excessive menstruation, simultaneous red and white vaginal discharge

Ingredients: Radix Albus Paeoniae Lactiflorae (*Bai Shao*), 100g, Radix Astragali Membranacei (*Huang Qi*), 100g, raw Radix Rehmanniae (*Sheng Di*), 100g, stir-fried Folium Artemisiae Argyii (*Ai Ye*), 30g

Method of preparation: Break up the above ingredients in a mortar to the size of large beans and then place in a large jar. Soak in 2 *jin* of alcohol and seal the lid. After 1 night it is ready for use.

Method of administration: Take warm before each meal any amount one wants.

Liu Ji Nu Jiu (Angelica Anomala Wine)

Functions: Breaks the blood and opens the channels, scatters stasis and stops pain

Mainly treats: Postpartum stasis, obstruction, and blood stagnation

Ingredients: Radix Angelicae Anomalae (*Liu Ji Nu*), Radix Glycyrrhizae (*Gan Cao*), equal parts

Method of preparation: Grind these 2 medicinals into a fine powder. Each time use 20g. First boil in 2 small teacups of water down to 1 small teacup. Then add 1 small teacup of alcohol and boil down again to 1 small teacup. Remove the dregs.

Method of administration: Take warm in 1 dose.

Dang Gui Di Huang Jiu (Dang Gui & Rehmannia Wine)

Functions: Supplements the blood, stops bleeding

Mainly treats: Postpartum uterine bleeding, abdominal pain

Ingredients: Raw Radix Rehmanniae (*Sheng Di*), 50g, Apex Radicis Angelicae Sinensis (*Dang Gui Wei*), 50g

Method of preparation: Grind the above 2 ingredients into a fine powder. Bring to a boil 100 times in 500g of yellow wine (*i.e.*, rice wine). Remove the dregs.

Method of administration: Take 20ml warm each time 3 times per day.

Da Bu Zhong Dang Gui Jiu (Greatly Supplementing the Center Dang Gui Wine)

Functions: Supplements vacuity detriment

Mainly treats: Postpartum vacuity detriment, lower abdominal aching and pain

Ingredients: Radix Angelicae Sinensis (*Dang Gui*), 40g, Radix Dipsaci (*Xu Duan*), 40g, Cortex Cinnamomi (*Rou Gui*), 40g, Rhizoma Ligustici Wallichii (*Chuan Xiong*), 40g, dry Rhizoma Zingiberis (*Gan Jiang*), 40g, Tuber Ophiopogonis Japonicae (*Mai Men Dong*), Radix Paeoniae Lactiflorae (*Shao Yao*), 60g, Fructus Evodiae Rutecarpae (*Wu Zhu Yu*), 100g, dry Radix Rehmanniae (*Gan Di Huang*), 100g, Radix Glycyrrhizae (*Gan Cao*), 30g, Radix Angelicae (*Bai Zhi*), 30g, Radix Astragali Membranacei (*Huang Qi*), 40g, Fructus Zizyphi Jujubae (*Da Zao*), 20 pieces

Method of preparation: Grind the above 13 medicinals into a fine powder and wrap in a cloth bag. Place in a large jar and soak in 4 *jin* of alcohol for 1 night. Then add 2 *jin* of water and boil down to 3 *jin* of liquid. Remove the dregs and store for use.

Method of administration: Take 15-20ml warm before each meal 3 times per day.

Hei Gui Jiu (Black Soybean & Cinnamon Wine)

Functions: Regulates the menses, warms the center, clears and eliminates cold and heat

Mainly treats: Postpartum qi and blood stasis and stagnation, generalized swelling and fullness, possible diarrhea or dysentery, alternating hot and cold

Ingredients: Stir-fried Semen Glycinis Hispidae (*Hei Dou*), 30g, Cortex Cinnamomi (*Rou Gui*), 30g, Radix Angelicae Sinensis (*Dang Gui*), 30g, Radix Paeoniae Lactiflorae (*Shao Yao*), 30g, blast-fried Rhizoma Zingiberis (*Pao Jiang*), 30g, raw Radix Rehmanniae (*Sheng Di*), 30g, mix-fried Radix Glycyrrhizae (*Zhi Gan Cao*), 20g, stir-fried Pollen Typhae (*Pu Huang*), 30g

Method of preparation: Grind the above 8 medicinals into a fine powder and place in a large jar. Soak in 3 *jin* for 7 nights. Then open, remove the dregs, and store for use.

Method of administration: Take 15-20ml 3 times per day.

181

Hong Lan Hua Jiu (Carthamus Wine)

Functions: Moves the blood, moistens dryness, disperses swelling, stops pain

Mainly treats: Women's wind stroke conditions, wind and cold invading the uterus, blood stasis and qi stagnation affecting the abdomen and causing piercing pain

Ingredients: Flos Carthami Tinctorii (*Hong Hua*), 30g

Method of preparation: Boil the above medicinal in 200ml of white alcohol until reduced by half. Remove the dregs and decant.

Method of administration: Take 50ml each time warm as needed.

Dang Gui Yuan Hu Jiu (Dang Gui & Corydalis Wine)

Functions: Quickens the blood and moves stasis

Mainly treats: Abdominal distention and pain accompanying the onset of the period

Ingredients: Radix Angelicae Sinensis (*Dang Gui*), 15g, Rhizoma Corydalis Yanhusuo (*Yan Hu Suo*), 15g, processed Myrrha (*Mo Yao*), 15g, Flos Carthami Tinctorii (*Hong Hua*), 15g

Method of preparation: Break up the above 4 ingredients in a mortar and place in a large jar. Soak in 2 *jin* of white alcohol. After 1 week open, remove the dregs, and store for use.

Method of administration: Take 1 teacup warm on an empty stomach morning and evening.

Mi Tang Huang Jiu (Honey & Rice Wine)

Functions: Nourishes the blood and moistens dryness

Mainly treats: Women's generalized itching

Ingredients: Honey (*Mi Tang*)

Method of preparation: Mix Honey with yellow (*i.e.*, rice) wine.

Method of administration: Drink a suitable amount at no fixed schedule.

10

Wines for Treating External Invasion & Damage by Wind

The wines in this chapter all treat the common cold, flu, and coughs in their initial stage accompanying the common cold. Because wine is upwardly and outwardly dispersing and resolves the exterior and because these conditions are located in the exterior according to TCM theory, these conditions can often be treated by medicinal wines no matter whether they are categorized as wind cold or wind heat. Also, because these conditions tend to come on rapidly, one can make such a wine beforehand and store it indefinitely until it is needed. Thus, one or more of these wines are useful to keep in one's home medicine closet.

Sang Ju Jiu (Morus & Chrysanthemum Wine)

Functions: Courses wind and clears heat, diffuses the lungs and stops coughing

Mainly treats: The initial stages of a wind warm condition with evils invading the upper burner, fever, slight aversion to wind and cold, cough, stuffy nose, slight oral thirst

Ingredients: Folium Mori Albi (*Sang Ye*), 30g, Flos Chrysanthemi Morifolii (*Ju Hua*), 30g, Herba Menthae (*Bo He*), 10g, Fructus Forsythiae Suspensae (*Lian Qiao*), Rhizoma Phragmitis Communis (*Lu Gen*), 35g, Semen Pruni Armeniacae (*Xing Ren*), 30g, Radix Platycodi Grandiflori (*Jie Geng*), 20g, Radix Glycyrrhizae (*Gan Cao*), 10g

Method of preparation: Grind the above 8 ingredients into a fine powder and place in a large jar. Soak in 2 *jin* of red rice wine and seal the lid. After 5 nights, open and store for use.

Method of administration: Take 15ml each time in the morning and evening.

Note: This is simply the tincture form of *Sang Ju Yin* (Morus & Chrysanthemum Drink).

Cong Chi Jiu (Allium & Fermented Soybean Wine)

Functions: Diffuses and opens the defensive qi, effuses and scatters wind and cold

Mainly treats: The initial stages of an external invasion, aversion to cold, fever, no sweating, headache, stuffed nose, bodily aches and vexation, chilly dysentery and abdominal pain

Ingredients: Herba Allii Fistulosi (*Cong Bai*), 3 roots, Semen Praeparatum Sojae (*Dan Dou Chi*), 15g

Method of preparation: Boil the above 2 medicinals in 300ml of alcohol until reduced by 1/2.

Method of administration: Take warm 2 times per day.

Man Jing Zi Jiu (Vitex Wine)

Functions: Courses and scatters wind heat, clears and disinhibits the head and eyes, stops pain

Mainly treats: External invasion of wind heat causing dizziness, headache, or one-sided headache

Ingredients: Fructus Viticis (*Man Jing Zi*), 200g

Method of preparation: Break up the above ingredient in a mortar and then place in a large jar. Soak in 1 *jin* of mellow wine and seal the lid. After 7 days, open the lid, remove the dregs, and store for use.

Method of administration: Take 10-15ml each time, 3 times per day.

Fu Fang Man Jing Zi Jiu (Compound Vitex Wine)

Functions: Courses wind, clears heat, stops pain

Mainly treats: Wind heat headache, dizziness, one-sided headache

Ingredients: Fructus Viticis (*Man Jing Zi*), 120g, Flos Chrysanthemi Morifolii (*Ju Hua*), 60g, Rhizoma Ligustici Wallichii (*Chuan Xiong*), 40g, Radix Ledebouriellae Sesloidis (*Fang Feng*), 60g, Herba Menthae (*Bo He*), 60g

Method of preparation: Break up the above medicinals in a mortar and place in a large jar. Soak in 2 *jin* of yellow wine (*i.e.*, rice wine) and seal the lid. After 7 days, open the lid, remove the dregs, and store for use.

Method of administration: Take 15ml each time, 3 times per day. One may increase this dose up to 20ml per time.

Jing Jie Chi Jiu (Schizonepeta & Fermented Soybean Wine)

Functions: Courses wind and disperses swelling

Mainly treats: External invasion of wind cold, fever, no sweating

Ingredients: Semen Praeparatum Sojae (*Dan Dou Chi*), 250g, Herba Seu Flos Schizonepetae Tenuifoliae (*Jing Jie*), 10g

Method of preparation: Place the above 2 ingredients in a large jar with 750ml of alcohol. Bring to a boil 5-7 times. Then remove the dregs and store for use.

Method of administration: Take warm each time as much as deemed appropriate.

11

Wines for Warding Off Scourges (*i.e.*, Pestilential Diseases)

Scourges refer to acute, communicable warm diseases which are pestilential in nature. Because the immune system in the elderly is typically depressed, they are more liable to catching any acute, seasonal, or epidemic disease. The wines in this chapter are meant to be taken by those living in an area currently in the grip of such an epidemic. As such, they can help prevent one from catching the disease that is going around.

Ku Shen Jiu (Sophora Wine)

Functions: Clears heat and resolves toxins, dispels miasmic qi

Mainly treats: Seasonal hot, toxic qi affecting the chest and diaphragm

Ingredients: Radix Sophorae Flavescentis (*Ku Shen*), 0.3g, Radix Platycodi Grandiflori (*Jie Geng*), 0.1g

Method of preparation: Grind the above 2 medicinals into a fine powder and place in a jar. Add 2 *jin* of alcohol and boil down to 1 *jin*. Remove the dregs and decant.

Method of administration: Take occasionally neither hot nor cold.

Jiang Zhi Jiu (Acronychia Stem Wine)

Functions: Wards off scourges

Mainly treats: Miasmic qi, wind damp foot qi

Ingredients: Ramulus Acronychiae Pedunculatae (*Jiang Cheng Xiang*), 60g, Fructus Zanthoxyli Bungeani (*Chuan Jiao*), 30g

Method of preparation: Place the above ingredients in a large jar and soak in 400ml of alcohol. After 7 days, open, remove the dregs, and store for use.

Method of administration: Take 10-15ml each time at no fixed schedule.

Tu Su Jiu (Reviving the Massacred Wine)

Functions: Wards off scourges and resolves toxic qi

Mainly treats: Miasmic qi, epidemics, pestilences, and all sorts of seasonal qi

Ingredients: Cortex Cinnamomi (*Rou Gui*), 23g, Radix Ledebouriellae Sesloidis (*Fang Feng*), 30g, Radix Platycodi Grandiflori (*Jie Geng*), 17g, Radix Et Rhizoma Rhei (*Da Huang*), 17g, processed Radix Aconiti (*Zhi Wu Tou*), 8g, Semen Phaseoli Calcarati (*Chi Xiao Dou*), 14 grains, Fructus Zanthoxyli Bungeani (*Shu Jiao*), 17g, Radix Smilacis Chinensis (*Ba Qia*), 15g

Method of preparation: Grind the above 8 medicinals into a fine powder and place in a large jar. Soak in 2 *jin* of alcohol and place this jar in a pan of water. Bring to a boil several times. Remove the dregs and store for use.

Method of administration: Take 1 teacup warm each morning on arising.

Sheng Niu Bang Gen Jiu (Fresh Burdock Root Wine)

Functions: Dispels miasmic qi

Mainly treats: Invasion of miasmic qi in tropical regions leading to flourishing of wind heat toxins in the human body, heart spirit vexation and oppression, foot and knee soreness and aching

Ingredients: Raw Radix Rehmanniae (*Sheng Di*), 30g, Radix Angelicae Pubescentis (*Du Huo*), 15g, Semen Glycinis Hispidae (*Hei Dou*), 100g, Cortex Erythrinae Variegatae (*Hai Tong Pi*), 30g, raw Radix Arctii Lappae (*Sheng Niu Bang Gen, i.e.*, Burdock root), 100g, Cortex Cinnamomi (*Rou Gui*), 15g, Semen Cannabis Sativae (*Huo Ma Ren*), 100g

Method of preparation: Grind the above 7 medicinals into a fine powder and place in a large jar. Soak in 3 *jin* of alcohol and seal the lid. After 3 days, open, remove the dregs, and store for use.

Method of administration: Take any amount one wishes warm before each meal.

191

Hua Tuo Bi Yi Jiu (Hua Tuo's Warding Off Epidemics Wine)

Functions: Wards off scourges and epidemics

Mainly treats: Invasions of tropical and mountain miasmic toxins

Ingredients: Radix Et Rhizoma Rhei (*Da Huang*), 15g, Rhizoma Atractylodis Macrocephalae (*Bai Zhu*), 15g, Cortex Cinnamomi (*Rou Gui*), 18g, Radix Platycodi Grandiflori (*Jie Geng*), 15g, Fructus Zanthoxyli Bungeani (*Shu Jiao*), 15g, Radix Aconiti (*Chuan Wu*), 6g, Radix Smilacis Chinensis (*Ba Qia*), 12g

Method of preparation: Place the above 7 medicinals in a large jar and hang this in the bottom of a well. After 10 days, take out. Then add 400ml of white alcohol and bring to a boil several times.

Method of administration: Take 1 small teacup each morning.

Jing Yue Tu Su Jiu (Jing-yue's Reviving the Massacred Wine)

Functions: Dispels wind dampness, wards off scourges and resolves toxins

Mainly treats: Mountain mist miasmic qi, scourges, epidemics, and seasonal qi

Ingredients: Herba Ephedrae (*Ma Huang*), 10g, Fructus Zanthoxyli Bungeani (*Chuan Jiao*), 10g, Herba Cum Radice Asari (*Xi Xin*), 10g, Radix Ledebouriellae Sesloidis (*Fang Feng*), 10g, Rhizoma Atractylodis (*Cang Zhu*), 10g, dry Rhizoma Zingiberis (*Gan Jiang*), 10g,

Cortex Cinnamomi (*Rou Gui*), 10g, Radix Platycodi Grandiflori (*Jie Geng*), 10g

Method of preparation: Grind the above 8 medicinals into a fine powder and place in a large jar. Soak in 2 *jin* of alcohol. After 5 days, open and store for use.

Method of administration: Take 1-2 small teacups on an empty stomach each day.

Contraindications: It is not appropriate to take too much of this wine.

12

Wines for Treating External Injuries

The wines in this chapter treat external injuries, such as contusions, strains, and sprains, from hitting, falling, and wrenching. The first three formulas treat more superficial injuries of the soft tissue which are characterized by their swelling and pain. The second three treat a deeper level of injury to the sinews and bones. These wines can be made in advance and kept in one's medicine closet for use when needed. The last two formulas both treat old traumatic injuries which have failed to heal.

Because Chinese medicinals which treat traumatic injuries mainly move the blood and dispel stasis and because such medicinals are contraindicated during pregnancy for fear of causing a miscarriage, the wines in this chapter should not be taken by pregnant women.

Su Mu Xing Yu Jiu (Sappan Moving Stasis Wine)

Functions: Moves the blood and dispels stasis, stops pain and disperses swelling

Mainly treats: Injuries due to hitting and falling, swelling and pain

Ingredients: Lignum Sappanis (*Su Mu*), 70g

Method of preparation: Grind the above ingredient into a fine powder and place in a large jar. Soak in 1 *jin* each of water and alcohol. Boil down to 1 *jin* and divide into 3 portions.

Method of administration: Take 1 portion on an empty stomach each morning, noon, and night.

Contraindications: Pregnant women should not take this formula.

Chuan Xiong Jiu (Ligusticum Wine)

Functions: Quickens the blood and stops pain

Mainly treats: Injury and damage due to fall and strike, one-sided headache

Ingredients: Rhizoma Ligustici Wallichii (*Chuan Xiong*), 90g

Method of preparation: Soak in 1kg of rice wine for 7 days.

Method of administration: Take 30g each time, 2 times per day.

Fo Shou Jiu (Buddha's Hand Wine)

Functions: Moves the qi and stops pain

Mainly treats: Aching and pain and internal injury due to fall or strike

Ingredients: Vinegar-processed Fructus Citri Sacrodactylis (*Fo Shou*), 15g

Method of preparation: Decoct the Fructus Citri Sacrodactylis in 30g of rice wine and a suitable amount of water.

Method of administration: Take warm 2 times per day.

Xu Jin Jie Gu Jiu (Extend the Sinews & Join the Bones Wine)

Functions: Joins the bones and extends the sinews, stops pain

Mainly treats: Falling and striking injuries

Ingredients: Herba Tougucao (*Tou Gu Cao*), 10g, Radix Et Rhizoma Rhei (*Da Huang*), 10g, Radix Angelicae Sinensis (*Dang Gui*), 10g, Radix Paeoniae Lactiflorae (*Shao Yao*), 10g, Cortex Radicis Moutan (*Dan Pi*), 6g, raw Radix Rehmanniae (*Sheng Di*), 15g, Gryllotalpa Africana (*Tu Gou*), 10 whole ones, Eupolyphaga Seu Opisthoplatia (*Tu Bie Chong*), 30 whole ones, Flos Carthami Tinctorii (*Hong Hua*), 10g, Pyritum (*Zi Ran Tong*), 3g

Method of preparation: Grind the first 9 medicinals above into a fine powder and place in a large jar. Boil in 350ml of alcohol until the liquid is reduced to 1/2. Remove the dregs and divide into 3 portions.

Method of administration: Take 1 portion warm each day chasing down the powdered Pyrite.

Contraindications: Pregnant women should not take this formula.

San Da Yao Jiu (Three Greats Medicinal Wine)

Functions: Quickens the blood and stabilizes pain, joins the bones and extends the sinews

Mainly treats: Detriment and damage due to falls and strikes, broken bones and damaged sinews

Ingredients: Radix Scopoliae Acutangulae (*San Fen San*), 2.5g, Herba Adhatodae Vasicae (*Da Bo Gu*), 2.5g, Pyritum (*Zi Ran Tong*), 2.5g, Lumbricus (*Di Long*), 2.5g, Fructus Immaturus Citri Seu Ponciri (*Zhi Shi*), 2.5g, Radix Paridis Petiolatae (*Chong Lou*), 2.5g, Fructus Piperis Nigri (*Hu Jiao*), 2.5g, Rhizoma Polygonati Cuspidati (*Hu Zhang*), 2.5g, processed Squama Manitis Pentadactylis (*Chuan Shan Jia*), 5g, Flos Carthami Tinctorii (*Hong Hua*), 5g, Sanguis Draconis (*Xue Jie*), 5g, Caulis Millettiae Seu Spatholobi (*Ji Xue Teng*), 5g, Ramus Loranthi Seu Visci (*Sang Ji Sheng*), 5g, Radix Achyranthis Bidentatae (*Niu Xi*), 5g, Rhizoma Ligustici Wallichii (*Chuan Xiong*), 5g, Radix Dipsaci (*Chuan Duan*), 5g

Method of preparation: Grind the above medicinals into a fine powder and wrap this in a cloth bag. Soak this in 500ml of alcohol for 48 hours or longer.

Method of administration: Drink 20-30ml each time, every 6 hours. Reduce this dosage for children.

Gu Sui Bu Jiu (Drynaria Wine)

Functions: Connects the bones and extends the sinews

Mainly treats: Injuries of the sinews and broken bones

Ingredients: Radix Drynariae (*Gu Sui Bu*), 720g

Method of preparation: Soak in 500g of yellow (*i.e.*, rice) wine for 7 days.

Method administration: Take 30ml each time, 2 times per day.

Huo Xue Jiu (Quicken the Blood Wine)

Functions: Opens the channels and quickens the blood

Mainly treats: Old traumatic injuries from hitting and falling, low back and lower leg pain due to cold dampness

Ingredients: Gummum Olibani (*Ru Xiang*), 15g, Myrrha (*Mo Yao*), 15g, Sanguis Draconis (*Xue Jie*), 15g, Bulbus Fritillariae (*Bei Mu*), 9g, Radix Et Rhizoma Notopterygii (*Qiang Huo*), 15g, Radix Saussureae Seu Vladimiriae (*Mu Xiang*), 6g, Cortex Magnoliae Officinalis (*Hou Po*), 9g, processed Radix Aconiti (*Zhi Chuan Wu*), 3g, processed Radix Aconiti (*Zhi Cao Wu*), 3g, Radix Angelicae (*Bai Zhi*), 24g, Secretio Moschi Moschiferi (*She Xiang*), 1.5g, Cortex Radicis Kadsurae (*Zi Jing Pi*), 24g, fresh Rhizoma Cyperi Rotundi (*Sheng Xiang Fu*), 15g, stir-fried Fructus Foeniculi Vulgaris (*Hui Xiang*), 9g, calcined Pyritum (*Zi Ran Tong*), 15g, Radix Angelicae Pubescentis (*Du Huo*), 15g, Radix Dipsaci (*Xu Duan*), 15g, Rhizoma Ligustici Wallichii (*Chuan Xiong*), 15g, Fructus Chaenomelis Lagenariae (*Mu Gua*), 15g, Cortex Cinnamomi (*Rou Gui*), 9g, Radix Angelicae Sinensis (*Dang Gui*), 24g

Method of preparation: Grind the above ingredients into a fine powder. Then wrap 15g of this powder in a cloth bag and soak in 500g of white alcohol for 7-10 days.

Method of administration: Drink a suitable amount at no fixed schedule.

Sun Shang Yao Jiu (Detriment & Damage Medicinal Wine)

Functions: Quickens the blood and soothes the sinews

199

Mainly treats: Many years old, persistent injury

Ingredients: Flos Carthami Tinctorii (*Hong Hua*), 6g, Radix Scutellariae Baicalensis (*Huang Qin*), 15g, Radix Linderae Strychnifoliae (*Wu Yao*), Sclerotium Poriae Cocos (*Fu Ling*), Radix Rehmanniae (*Sheng Di*), 15g, Cortex Radicis Acanthopanacis (*Wu Jia Pi*), 15g, Cortex Eucommiae Ulmoidis (*Du Zhong*), 15g, Radix Achyranthis Bidentatae (*Niu Xi*), 15g, Radix Polygalae Tenuifoliae (*Yuan Zhi*), 15g, Tuber Ophiopogonis Japonicae (*Mai Men Dong*), 15g, Radix Gentianae Macrophyllae (*Qin Jiao*), 15g, Cortex Radicis Moutan (*Dan Pi*), 15g, Nodus Pini (*Song Jie*), 15g, Rhizoma Alismatis (*Ze Xie*), 15g, Rhizoma Corydalis Yanhusuo (*Yan Hu Suo*), 15g, Radix Angelicae Sinensis (*Dang Gui*), 18g, Fructus Lycii Chinensis (*Gou Qi Zi*), 18g, Semen Pruni Persicae (*Tao Ren*), 12g, Gelatinum Corii Asini (*E Jiao*), 12g, Radix Dipsaci (*Xu Duan*), 9g, Fructus Psoraleae Corylifoliae (*Bu Gu Zhi*), 9g, Fructus Citri Seu Ponciri (*Zhi Qiao*), 9g, Ramulus Cinnamomi (*Gui Zhi*), Rhizoma Cyperi Rotundi (*Xiang Fu*), 9g

Method of preparation: Soak in an appropriate amount of alcohol for at least 7 days.

Method of administration: Take 1 small teacup per day.

13

Wines for Treating Herpes Zoster & Other Skin Lesions

In Chinese, *pao zhen* means blistery skin lesions in general and herpes zoster in particular. Herpes zoster is typically seen in the elderly, the weak, or the chronically ill. It is a chronic viral disease which lies latent until the host immune system becomes weakened. In such cases, the virus is then able to become active and moves toward the surface, following the pathways of the nerves. A number of the formulas in this chapter treat herpes zoster. Herpes is usually a damp hot condition, and, therefore, alcohol can actually cause this problem in a patient who is not used to drinking alcohol or who has drunk more than their usual amount. Nonetheless, when combined with the appropriate ingredients, medicated wines can also treat this problem.

Other formulas in this chapter treat *yong* and *ju* and other stubborn, recalcitrant skin diseases, such as eczema and psoriasis. Since most of these skin diseases contain a component of blood stasis, the alcohol in these formulas helps to move the blood and dispel stasis.

Zhi Qiao Qin Jiao Jiu (Citrus & Gentiana Macrophylla Wine)

Functions: Courses wind and stops itching, recedes rashes

Mainly treats: Itchy skin rashes which feel as if insects were moving in them

Ingredients: Fructus Citri Seu Ponciri (*Zhi Qiao*), 90g, Radix Gentiana Macrophyllae (*Qin Jiao*), 120g, Radix Salviae Miltiorrhizae (*Dan Shen*), 150g, Radix Angelicae Pubescentis (*Du Huo*), 120g, Herba Cistanchis (*Rou Cong Rong*), 120g, Caulis Et Folium Sambucudis Javanicae (*Lu Ying*), 100g, Folium Pini (*Song Ye, i.e.*, pine needles), 250g

Method of preparation: Pestle the above medicinals into pieces and place in a large jar. Soak in 4 *jin* of white alcohol and seal the lid. After 7 days, open, remove the dregs, and store for use.

Method of administration: Take 10-15ml each time, 3 times per day. One may increase this dose up to 20ml.

Niu Bang Chan Tui Jiu (Arctium & Periostracum Cicadae Wine)

Functions: Scatters wind and diffuses the lungs, clears heat and resolves toxins, disinhibits the throat and scatters nodulation, recedes rashes

Mainly treats: Swelling and pain of the throat, cough, itching, vomiting of phlegm, measles, urticaria

Ingredients: Fructus Arctii Lappae (*Niu Bang Zi*), 1 *jin*, Periostracum Cicadae (*Chan Tui*), 30g

Method of preparation: Soak the above 2 ingredients in 3 *jin* of alcohol. After 3 days, open the lid and remove the dregs.

Method of administration: Take 1-2 teacups after each meal.

Contraindications: This formula is not appropriate for those with spleen/stomach cold damp diarrhea.

Niu Bang Di Huang Jiu (Arctium & Rehmannia Wine)

Functions: Clears heat and resolves toxins, nourishes yin and cools the blood, boosts the liver and kidneys

Mainly treats: Wind toxin blisters and *yong* which do not heal, slackness and weakness of the four limbs, soreness and fatigue of the low back and knees

Ingredients: Fructus Arctii Lappae (*Niu Bang Zi*), 100g, raw Radix Rehmanniae (*Sheng Di*), 100g, Fructus Lycii Chinensis (*Gou Qi Zi*), 100g, Radix Achyranthis Bidentatae (*Niu Xi*), 20g

Method of preparation: Grind the above 4 ingredients and place them in a large jar. Soak in 3 *jin* of alcohol and seal the lid. Allow to tincture for 7 days in the spring and summer and for 14 days in the fall and winter. Then open and remove the dregs.

Method of administration: Take 1-2 teacups each time, warm on an empty stomach after the evening meal. It is good to feel a little tipsy.

Huai Hua Jiu (Sophora Flower Wine)

Functions: Resolves toxins, eliminates wind, cools the blood

Mainly treats: Toxic blisters which have or have not yet fully developed

Ingredients: Flos Immaturus Sophorae Japonicae (*Huai Hua*), 120g

Method of preparation: Stir-fry the Flos Sophorae until yellow and then soak in 500ml of yellow wine (*i.e.*, rice wine). Bring to a boil 10 times and then remove the dregs. Store for use.

Method of administration: Take hot to induce sweating. If the blisters have not yet already fully developed, take 2-3 times. If the blisters have already fully developed, take 1-2 times.

Shi Nan Fu Zi Jiu (Photinia & Kochia Wine)

Functions: Eliminates wind dampness, harmonizes the blood and stops itching

Mainly treats: Wind toxin measles rash

Ingredients: Folium Photiniae Serrulatae (*Shi Nan Ye*), 50g, Fructus Kochiae Scopariae (*Di Fu Zi*), 50g, Radix Angelicae Sinensis (*Dang Gui*), 50g, Radix Angelicae Pubescentis (*Du Huo*), 50g

Method of preparation: Grind the above medicinals into a fine powder and store for use.

Method of administration: Use 5-6g of the above powder each time in 1 teacup of alcohol (approximately 15ml) and bring to a boil several times. Take 3 times per day on an empty stomach.

Jin Yin Hua Jiu (Lonicera Wine)

Functions: Clears heat and resolves toxins

Mainly treats: Blistery swollen rashes, lung *yong*, intestinal *yong*

Ingredients: Flos Lonicerae Japonicae (*Jin Yin Hua*), 50g, Radix Glycyrrhizae (*Gan Cao*), 10g

Method of preparation: Boil the above 2 medicinals in 2 bowls of water down to 1/2 bowl. Then add 1/2 bowl of alcohol and briefly boil again. Divide into 3 portions.

Method of administration: Take 1 portion each morning, noon, and night.

Gua Lou Gan Cao Jiu (Trichosanthes & Licorice Wine)

Functions: Disperses swelling, transforms stasis

Mainly treats: Chronic *yong* and clove sores which do not heal after many days

Ingredients: Fructus Trichosanthis Kirlowii (*Gua Lou*), 1 piece, Radix Glycyrrhizae (*Gan Cao*), 2g

Method of preparation: Grind the above 2 ingredients into a fine powder. Use 1 small teacup of water and 1 small teacup of wine. Bring to a boil 3-5 times and remove the dregs.

Method of administration: Take warm as needed.

Jin Xing Gan Cao Jiu (Phymatopsis & Licorice Wine)

Functions: Disperses swelling and stops pain

Mainly treats: Toxic swellings erupting on the upper back

Ingredients: Herba Phymatopsis Griffithianae (*Jin Xing Cao*), 50g, Radix Glycyrrhizae (*Gan Cao*), 3g

Method of preparation: Grind the above 2 medicinals into a fine powder and place in a large jar. Soak in 1 *jin* of alcohol and open after 7 days.

Method of administration: Take a little bit, little bit at no fixed schedule.

Fu Fang Hong Hua Jiu (Compound Carthamus Wine)

Functions: Quickens the blood and transforms stasis, disperses swelling and stops pain, clears heat and resolves toxins, closes ulcers and promotes the growth of new flesh

Mainly treats: Bedsores

Ingredients: Flos Carthami Tinctorii (*Hong Hua*), 50g, Radix Astragali Membranacei (*Huang Qi*), 30g, Radix Ampelopsis (*Bai Lian*), 20g

Method of preparation: Add these medicinals to 500ml of 75% alcohol and allow to soak for 7 nights. then remove the dregs and store for use.

Method of administration: Apply externally to the affected area.

Shen Xiao Jiu (Divinely Efficacious Wine)

Functions: Expels toxins, scatters toxins

Mainly treats: Blistery rashes and *yong*

Ingredients: Radix Panacis Ginseng (*Ren Shen*), 30g, Myrrha (*Mo Yao*), 30g, Apex Radicis Angelicae Sinensis (*Dang Gui Wei*), 30g, Radix Glycyrrhizae (*Gan Cao*), 15g, Fructus Trichosanthis Kirlowii (*Gua Lou*), 1 piece

Method of preparation: Place the above medicinals in 3 bowls of yellow wine (*i.e.*, rice wine) and boil down to 2 bowls of liquid. Then divide into 4 portions.

Method of administration: Take 1 portion each day, little bit, little bit at a time.

Shou Wu Chuan Shan Jia Jiu (Polygonum Multiflorum & Squama Manitis Wine)

Functions: Dispels wind and resolves toxins

Mainly treats: Ox skin *xian* (*i.e.*, psoriasis)

Ingredients: Radix Polygoni Multiflori (*Shou Wu*), 30g, Radix Angelicae Sinensis (*Dang Gui*), 20g, Squama Manitis Pentadactylae (*Chuan Shan Jia*), 20g, raw Radix Rehmanniae (*Sheng Di*), 20g, prepared Radix Rehmanniae (*Shu Di*), 20g, Rana Limnocharis (*Ha Ma, i.e.*, a species of toad), 20g, Cacumen Biotae Orientalis (*Ce Bai Ye*), 15g, Folium Pini (*Song Zhen, i.e.*, Pine Needles), 30g, Cortex Radicis Acanthopanacis (*Wu Jia Pi*), Radix Aconiti (*Chuan Wu & Cao Wu*), each 5g

Method of preparation: Grind the above 10 ingredients into a fine powder and place in a large jar. Soak in 6 *jin* of yellow wine (*i.e.*, rice wine) and seal the lid. After 7 days, open, remove the dregs, and store for use.

Method of administration: Take warm on an empty stomach whatever amount one wishes at no fixed schedule.

Zhi Qiao Dan Shen Jiu (Citrus & Salvia Wine)

Functions: Courses wind and stops pain

Mainly treats: Wind itching, the feeling as if insects were moving in the skin

Ingredients: Fructus Citri Seu Ponciri (*Zhi Qiao*), 18g, Radix Gentianae Macrophyllae (*Qin Jiao*), 15g, Radix Angelicae Pubescentis (*Du Huo*), Herba Cistanchis (*Rou Cong Rong*), 15g, Radix Salviae Miltiorrhizae (*Dan Shen*), 18g, Caulis Et Folium Sambucudis Javanicae (*Lu Ying*), 18g, Folium Pini (*Song Ye*), 50g

Method of preparation: Grind the above 7 ingredients into a fine powder and place in a large jar. Soak in 2 *jin* of clear alcohol and seal the lid. After 7 days, open the lid, remove the dregs, and store for use.

Method of administration: Take any amount one wishes warm at no fixed schedule.

Song Ye Jiu (Pine Needle Wine)

Functions: Dispels wind, stops itching, resolves toxins

Mainly treats: Urticaria and measles rash

Ingredients: Folium Pini (*Song Ye*), 1 *jin*

Method of preparation: Cut up into small pieces and put in 2 *jin* of alcohol. Boil down to 300ml and remove the dregs.

Method of administration: Each evening, drink a moderate amount warm. Sweating results in a cure.

Gan Cao Sheng Ma Jiu (Licorice & Cimicifuga Wine)

Functions: Disperses swelling and stops pain

Mainly treats: Toxic swellings on the head and upper body, piercing pain difficult to bear

Ingredients: Mix-fried Radix Glycyrrhizae (*Zhi Gan Cao*), 20g, Rhizoma Cimicifugae (*Sheng Ma*), 20g, Lignum Aquilariae Agallochae (*Chen Xiang*), 20g, Secretio Moschi Moschiferi (*She Xiang*), 0.6g, Semen Praeparatum Sojae (*Dan Dou Chi*), 36g

Method of preparation: Grind the above ingredients, excepting the Musk, into a fine powder. Then mix in the powdered Musk and store in a sealed jar.

Method of administration: Each time, boil 15g of the above powder in 1 teacup of alcohol and reduce the liquid to 8/10. Remove the dregs. Take 1 time each morning and evening before meals. Also apply the dregs hot to the swollen area.

Fu She Jiu (Agkistrodon Wine)

Functions: Dispels wind and resolves toxins

209

Mainly treats: Psoriasis

Ingredients: Agkistrodon Acutus (*Fu She*), 1 strip, Radix Panacis Ginseng (*Ren Shen*), 15g

Method of preparation: Place the dried snake and Ginseng in a large jar and soak in 2 *jin* of alcohol. After 7 days, open and store for use.

Method of administration: Take whatever amount one wishes at no fixed schedule.

Ban Mao Jiu (Mylabris Wine)

Functions: Attacks toxins, disperses sores

Mainly treats: Alopecia areata

Ingredients: Mylabris (*Ban Mao*), 15 whole ones

Method of preparation: Grind the above ingredient and place it in a large jar. Soak in 200ml of alcohol. After 5 days, open and store for use.

Method of administration: Apply to the affected area 2 times per day.

Contraindications: Do not take internally, since it is toxic when done so.

Jie Du Xiao Pao Jiu (Resolve Toxins, Disperse Sores Wine)

Functions: Dispels wind and resolves toxins

Mainly treats: Plum sores, wind toxin low back pain

Ingredients: Radix Achyranthis Bidentatae (*Niu Xi*), 30g, Rhizoma Ligustici Wallichii (*Chuan Xiong*), 30g, Radix Et Rhizoma Notopterygii (*Qiang Huo*), Cortex Radicis Acanthopanacis (*Wu Jia Pi*), 30g, Cortex Eucommiae Ulmoidis (*Du Zhong*), 30g, Radix Glycyrrhizae (*Gan Cao*), 30g, Cortex Radicis Lycii (*Di Gu Pi*), 30g, Semen Coicis Lachryma-jobi (*Yi Yi Ren*), 30g, raw Radix Rehmanniae (*Sheng Di*), 200g, Cortex Erythrinae Variegatae (*Hai Tong Pi*), 60g

Method of preparation: Grind the above medicinals into a fine powder and place in a large jar. Soak in 4 *jin* of alcohol. Allow to tincture 5 days in the spring and summer and for 10 days in the fall and winter. Then open the lid, remove the dregs, and store for use.

Method of administration: Take 10-15ml before meals, 3 times per day.

He Shou Wu Jiu (Polygonum Multiflorum Wine)

Function: Enriches the constructive and disperses toxins

Mainly treats: Numbness wind of leprosy manifesting some slight vacuity symptoms

Ingredients: Radix Polygoni Multiflori (*He Shou Wu*), 120g, Radix Angelicae Sinensis (*Dang Gui*), 30g, Apex Radicis Angelicae Sinensis (*Dang Gui Wei*), 30g, mix-fried Squama Manitis (*Chuan Shan Jia*),

211

30g, Radix Rehmanniae (*Sheng Di*), 30g, prepared Radix Rehmanniae (*Shu Di*), 30g, Rana Limnocharis (*Ha Ma*), 30g, Cacumen Biotae Orientalis (*Ce Bai Ye*), 12g, Folium Pini (*Song Zhen, i.e.,* Pine Needles), 12g, Cortex Radicis Acanthopanacis (*Wu Jia Pi*), 12g, processed Radix Aconiti (*Zhi Cao Wu*), 12g

Method of preparation: Place the above medicinals in a large jar and soak in 10 *jin* of yellow (*i.e.,* rice) wine. Seal the lid. Allow to tincture for at least 10 days.

Method of administration: Depending on the severity of the condition, take either more or less of this wine. Drink until one begins to sweat.

Contraindications: Do not expose oneself to wind when sweating due to drinking this wine.

Lou Tong Jiu (Rhaponticus Opening Wine)

Functions: Opens the channels and network vessels

Mainly treats: The initial stages of breast abscess

Ingredients: Radix Rhapontici Seu Echinopsis (*Lou Lu*), 10g, Caulis Akebiae Mutong (*Mu Tong*), 10g, Bulbus Fritillariae Cirrhosae (*Chuan Bei Mu*), 10g, Radix Glycyrrhizae (*Gan Cao*), 6g

Method of preparation: Place the above ingredients in 1 large teacup apiece of water and wine (*i.e.,* a total of 2 teacupsful) and boil down to 1 teacup. Remove the dregs and divide into 2 portions.

Method of administration: Take 1 portion warm after meals in the evening.

Gong Jin Jiu (Dandelion & Lonicera Wine)

Functions: Clears heat and resolves toxins

Mainly treats: Mastitis

Ingredients: Herba Taraxaci Mongolici (*Pu Gong Ying*), 15g, Flos Lonicerae Japonicae (*Jin Yin Hua*), 15g

Method of preparation: Place the Taraxacum and Lonicera in 2 teacups of yellow wine (*i.e.*, rice wine) and boil down to 1/2 the amount of liquid. Remove the dregs and divide into 2 portions.

Method of administration: Take 1 portion after meals morning and night. Also apply the dregs to the affected area.

14

Miscellaneous Wines

The medicinal wines in this chapter treat a number of different conditions. These include lung problems, vision problems, parasites, thromboangiitis obliterans, lateral costal pain, lower abdominal distention and fullness, etc.

Ma Huang Xuan Fei Jiu (Ephedra Diffusing the Lungs Wine)

Functions: Diffuses depressed qi in the lungs

Mainly treats: Acne rosacea or brandy nose

Ingredients: Herba Ephedrae (*Ma Huang*), 30g, Radix Ephedrae (*Ma Huang Gen*), 30g

Method of preparation: Soak the above medicinals in 1 *jin* of white alcohol and then decoct for approximately 1 hour. Allow to sit over night and then remove the dregs. Store for use.

Method of administration: Take 2-3 small teacups morning and night.

Note: After taking 1, 3, or 5 days, one will spit up some purulent pus. After 10 days, this pus will be exhausted. Then there will be some red colored phlegm. This should give way to yellow and thence to white colored phlegm. When this occurs, one will be cured.

Sang Bai Pi Jiu (Cortex Mori Wine)

Functions: Stabilizes wheezing

Mainly treats: Lung heat coughing and wheezing

Ingredients: Cortex Radicis Mori (*Sang Bai Pi*), 200g

Method of preparation: Cut the Morus into pieces and place in a large jar. Soak in 1kg of rice wine for 7 days.

Method of administration: Take 20ml each time, 3 times per day.

Zi Su Zi Jiu (Perilla Seed Wine)

Functions: Downbears counterflow, transforms phlegm, and stops coughing and wheezing

Mainly treats: Phlegm congelation obstruction and blockage, lung qi upward counterflow resulting in wheezing

Ingredients: Fructus Perillae Frutescentis (*Zi Su Zi*), 600g

Method of preparation: Slightly stir-fry the Perilla Seeds and then soak them in 2.5kg of yellow (*i.e.*, rice) wine for 7 days.

Method of administration: Take 10ml each time, 2 times per day.

Gua Lou Xie Bai Jiu (Trichosanthes & Allium Macrostemon Wine)

Functions: Opens yang and scatters nodulation, moves the qi and dispels phlegm

Mainly treats: Shortness of breath, chest and upper back pain, wheezing and panting, coughing saliva

Ingredients: Fructus Trichosanthis Kirlowii (*Gua Lou*), 1 piece, Bulbus Allii (*Xie Bai*), 60g

Method of preparation: Place the above 2 ingredients in 300ml of rice wine. Decoct down to 200ml.

Method of administration: Take 1-2 small teacups warm each time, 1 time per day.

Hu Lu Jiu (Bottle Gourd Wine)

Functions: Opens the portals

Mainly treats: Stuffed nose, eye pain and dimming of vision, brain oppression

Ingredients: Semen Lagenariae Sicerariae (*Ku Hu Lu Zi*), 30g

Method of preparation: Soak the above seeds in 150ml of mellow wine. After 7 days, open the lid and remove the dregs. Store for use.

Method of administration: Little bit, little bit, snuffle this wine up the nose 3-4 times per day. (One can also use a nose dropper.)

Bai Bu Jiu (Stemona Wine)

Functions: Moistens the lungs and descends the qi, stops coughing and kills worms (*i.e.*, parasites)

Mainly treats: Cough, rapid breathing, hundred day cough (*i.e.*, whooping cough), bronchitis, etc. When used externally, this wine kills parasites and treats scabies, vaginal trichomoniasis and hemophilus, etc.

Ingredients: Radix Stemonae (*Bai Bu*), 100g

Method of preparation: Soak the Stemona in 500ml of white alcohol. After 7 days, open and remove the dregs. Then store for use.

Method of administration: Take 15ml after meals, 3 times per day. Externally, apply to the affected area.

Contraindications: Do not use in case of spleen/stomach vacuity weakness or diarrhea.

Tong Mai Guan Yao Jiu (Opening the Blood Vessels Medicinal Wine)

Functions: Quickens the blood and opens the vessels, transforms stasis and stops pain

Mainly treats: Thromboangiitis obliterans due to qi stagnation, blood stasis tending to cold

Ingredients: Rhizoma Paridis Polyphyllae (*Qi Ye Yi Zhi Hua*), 30g, Rhizoma Ardisiae (*Zou Ma Tai*), 30g, Apex Radicis Angelicae Sinensis (*Dang Gui Wei*), 30g, Ramus Loranthi Seu Visci (*Sang Ji*

Sheng), 30g, Radix Clematidis Chinensis (*Wei Ling Xian*), 30g, Radix Achyranthis Bidentatae (*Niu Xi*), 15g, Ramulus Cinnamomi (*Gui Zhi*), 15g, Flos Carthami Tinctorii (*Hong Hua*), 15g, Semen Pruni Persicae (*Tao Ren*), 15g, Spinae Gleditschiae Chinensis (*Zao Jiao Ci*), 15g, Gummum Olibani (*Ru Xiang*), 9g, Myrrha (*Mo Yao*), 9g, Radix Astragali Membranacei (*Huang Qi*), 15g, Radix Codonopsis Pilosulae (*Dang Shen*), 15g

Method of preparation: Soak the above medicinals in 5-6 *jin* of yellow (*i.e.*, rice) wine for 3 weeks.

Method of administration: Take 20-100ml each time, 4-6 times per day. However, do not get drunk. One month equals 1 course of treatment.

Zhu Yu Gen Jiu (Evodia Root Wine)

Functions: Expels worms (*i.e.*, parasites)

Mainly treats: Spleen vacuity heat, vomiting, and discharge of worms

Ingredients: Radix Evodiae Rutecarpae (*Wu Zhu Yu Gen*), 1/2 foot of a large root, Semen Cannabis Sativae (*Huo Ma Ren*), 50g, Pericarpium Citri Reticulatae (*Chen Pi*), 25g

Method of preparation: Pestle these 3 ingredients into pieces and place in a large jar. Soak in 2 *jin* of yellow (*i.e.*, rice) wine. After 1 night, cook over a small fire. Then remove the dregs and store for use.

Method of administration: Take 1-2 small teacups on an empty stomach each morning and before eating in the evening. When worms are discharged below, stop taking.

Ku Shen Jie Du Jiu (Sophora Resolve Toxins Wine)

Functions: Resolves toxins

Mainly treats: Food poisoning

Ingredients: Radix Sophorae Flavescentis (*Ku Shen*), 45g

Method of preparation: Decoct the Sophora in 500ml of good alcohol down to 250ml. Remove the dregs and use warm.

Method of administration: Having drunk whatever amount, vomiting results in a cure.

Qin Jiao Jiu (Gentiana Macrophylla Wine)

Functions: Dispels wind cold, stops pain, opens the two excretions

Mainly treats: Lower abdominal distention and fullness, aching and pain refusing pressure, astringent, inhibited urination, defecation not open, runny nose with clear snivel

Ingredients: Radix Gentianae Macrophyllae (*Qin Jiao*), 30g, Radix Achyranthis Bidentatae (*Niu Xi*), 30g, Rhizoma Ligustici Wallichii (*Chuan Xiong*), 30g, Radix Ledebouriellae Sesloidis (*Fang Feng*), 30g, Cortex Eucommiae Ulmoidis (*Du Zhong*), 30g, Sclerotium Rubrum Poriae Cocos (*Chi Fu Ling*), 30g, Radix Salviae Miltiorrhizae (*Dan Shen*), 30g, Radix Angelicae Pubescentis (*Du Huo*), 30g, Cortex

Radicis Lycii (*Di Gu Pi*), 30g, Semen Coicis Lachryma-jobi (*Yi Yi Ren*), 30g, Semen Cannabis Sativae (*Huo Ma Ren*), 30g, Cortex Cinnamomi (*Rou Gui*), 25g, Herba Dendrobii (*Shi Hu*), 20g, dry Rhizoma Zingiberis (*Gan Jiang*), 20g, Cortex Radicis Acanthopanacis (*Wu Jia Pi*), 50g, Radix Praeparatus Aconiti Carmichaeli (*Zhi Fu Zi*), 24g, Tuber Ophiopogonis Japonicae (*Mai Men Dong*), 25g

Method of preparation: Grind the above 17 ingredients into a fine powder and place in a large jar. Soak in 3 *jin* of alcohol for 5 days in the spring and summer and for 7 days in the fall and winter. Then open and remove the dregs.

Method of administration: Take 10-20ml warm on an empty stomach each day. When cured, stop.

Huo Ma Ren Jiu (Cannabis Wine)

Functions: Moistens the intestines and opens the bowels while simultaneously supplementing the center

Mainly treats: Geriatric constipation, women's postpartum constipation, and constipation due to the aftermath of a hot disease with blood vacuity and scanty fluids and humors, lower abdominal distention, fullness, aching, and pain accompanied by constipation

Ingredients: Stir-fried till fragrant Semen Cannabis Sativae (*Huo Ma Ren*), 160g

Method of preparation: Grind the above ingredient into a fine powder and soak in 500ml of good alcohol. After 3 nights, open and remove the dregs.

Method of administration: Take a suitable amount warm each time before each meal, but do not get drunk.

Tao Ren Jiu (Persica Wine)

Functions: Moistens the intestines and opens the bowels

Mainly treats: Postpartum blood vacuity constipation

Ingredients: Semen Pruni Persicae (*Tao Ren*), 60g

Method of preparation: Smash the above ingredient and soak in 1kg of rice wine for 10 days.

Method of administration: Take 30ml each time, 2 times per day.

Cang Er Jiu (Xanthium Wine)

Functions: Eliminates heat, supplements vacuity

Mainly treats: Bone aching, tinnitus

Ingredients: Fructus Xanthii (*Cang Er Zi*), 30g, Radix Ledebouriellae Sesloidis (*Fang Feng*), 30g, stir-fried Fructus Arctii Lappae (*Niu Bang Zi*), 30g, Radix Rehmanniae (*Sheng Di*), 30g, Caulis Akebiae Mutong (*Mu Tong*), 20g, Radix Astragali Membranacei (*Huang Qi*), 30g, Sclerotium Poriae Cocos (*Fu Ling*), 30g, Radix Angelicae Pubescentis (*Du Huo*), 30g, Semen Coicis Lachryma-jobi (*Yi Yi Ren*), 20g, Radix Panacis Ginseng (*Ren Shen*), 15g, Cortex Cinnamomi (*Rou Gui*), 12g

Method of preparation: Pestle the above 11 ingredients and place them in a large jar. Soak in 2 *jin* of alcohol and seal the lid. After 7 days, open and remove the dregs.

Method of administration: Take 1-2 small teacups each day on an empty stomach. One can increase this dose as necessary to 2-3 small teacups.

Chang Pu Gui Xin Jiu (Acorus & Cinnamon Wine)

Functions: Opens the portals and dispels wind, promotes qi absorption and subdues yang, quiets the spirit

Mainly treats: Tinnitus and deafness

Ingredients: Rhizoma Acori Graminei (*Shi Chang Pu*), 2g, Caulis Akebiae Mutong (*Mu Tong*), 1g, Cortex Cinnamomi (*Gui Xin*), 15g, Magnetitum (*Ci Shi*), 15g, Radix Ledebouriellae Sesloidis (*Fang Feng*), 30g, Radix Et Rhizoma Notopterygii (*Qiang Huo*), 30g

Method of preparation: Grind the above 6 ingredients into a coarse powder and place in a cloth bag. Put this in a large jar and soak on 1 *jin* of alcohol for 7 days. Then remove the dregs and store for use.

Method of administration: Take 10-20ml warm on an empty stomach each day.

Ci Shi Jiu (Magnetite Wine)

Functions: Opens the portals, promotes the absorption of qi and subdues yang

223

Mainly treats: Liver/kidney yin vacuity leading to deafness and tinnitus

Ingredients: Magnetitum (*Ci Shi*), 15g, Caulis Akebiae Mutong (*Mu Tong*), 250g, Rhizoma Acori Graminei (*Shi Chang Pu*), 250g

Method of preparation: Grind the above 3 ingredients into a coarse powder and place in a cloth bag. Then place this in a large jar and soak in 2 *jin* of alcohol. Seal the lid and allow to tincture for 3 days in the summer and 7 days in the winter. Remove the dregs and store for use.

Method of administration: Take 1-2 small teacups after each meal.

Fo Shou Jiu (Buddha's Hand Wine)

Functions: Nourishes the center and harmonizes the stomach

Mainly treats: Stomach reflux and choking of the diaphragm (*i.e.*, cancer of the esophagus)

Ingredients: Fructus Citri Sacrodactylis (*Fo Shou*), 30g, dried Semen Eleocharis Tuberosae (*Bi Qi, i.e.*, Water Chestnut), 30g, Semen Nelumbinis Nuciferae (*Lian Zi Rou*), 30g, Fructus Zizyphi Jujubae (*Da Zao*), 30g, Semen Coicis Lachryma-jobi (*Yi Yi Ren*), 30g, Cortex Cinnamomi (*Rou Gui*), 30g, dry Fructus Diospyros Kaki (*Shi Bing, i.e.*, Persimmon), 30g, Fructus Canarii (*Gan Lan*), 30g

Method of preparation: Soak the above 8 medicinals in 5 *jin* of roasted barley alcohol. After 7 days, open, remove the dregs, and store for use.

Method of administration: Take 1-2 small teacups warm on an empty stomach each time, 3 times per day.

Mei Gui Hua Jiu (Rosa Rugosa Wine)

Functions: Courses the liver and rectifies the qi, harmonizes the stomach and stops pain

Mainly treats: Liver/stomach qi pain, menstrual irregularity, abnormal vaginal discharge

Ingredients: Flos Rosae Rugosae (*Mei Gui Hua*), 30g

Method of preparation: Soak the above medicinal in 500g of rice wine for 1/2 month.

Method of administration: Take 20ml each time, 2 times per day.

Gui Hua Jiu (Osmanthus Flower Wine)

Functions: Transforms phlegm and scatters stasis

Mainly treats: Liver/stomach qi pain and abdominal distention

Ingredients: Flos Osmanthi Fragrantis (*Gui Hua*), 60g

Method of preparation: Soak the above ingredient in 500g of rice wine for 15 days.

Method of administration: Take 30ml each time, 2 times per day.

Ju Pi Jiu (Orange Peel Wine)

Functions: Rectifies the qi and opens the stomach

Mainly treats: Vomiting and nausea, reduced appetite, abdominal distention

Ingredients: Pericarpium Citri Reticulatae (*Ju Pi*), 60g

Method of preparation: Grind the Orange Peel into powder and soak in 1kg of rice wine for 10 days.

Method of administration: Take 30ml each time, 2 times per day.

Ju Hua Jiu (Chrysanthemum Wine)

Functions: Clears liver heat, brightens the eyes

Mainly treats: Dizziness, headache, red eyes, blurred vision

Ingredients: Flos Chrysanthemi Morifolii (*Bai Ju Hua*), 60g

Method of preparation: Cut the Chrysanthemum into pieces and soak in 500ml of rice wine for 7 days.

Method of administration: Take 30ml each time, 2 times per day.

Wu Wei Zi Jiu (Schizandra Wine)

Functions: Calms the heart and quiets the spirit

Mainly treats: Insomnia

Ingredients: Fructus Schizandrae Chinensis (*Wu Wei Zi*), 150g

Method of preparation: Soak the Schizandra in 500ml of white alcohol for 1 month.

Method of administration: Take 15g each time, 3 times per day.

Ting Xin Jiu (Tranquilize the Heart Wine)

Functions: Tranquilizes the heart

Mainly treats: Insomnia, poor memory

Ingredients: Arillus Euphoriae Longanae (*Long Yan Rou*), 500g, Flos Osmanthi Fragrantis (*Gui Hua*), 120g, White Sugar (*Bai Tang*), 240g

Method of preparation: Place the above 3 medicinals in a large jar and soak in 5kg of white alcohol for 1/2 month.

Method of administration: Take whatever amount one wishes at no fixed schedule. However, do not get drunk.

Hai Zao Jiu (Sargassium Wine)

Functions: Transforms phlegm and scatters nodulation

Mainly treats: Benign hypertrophy of the thyroid, insufficient thyroid function

Ingredients: Herba Sargassii (*Hai Zao*), 500g

Method of preparation: Soak the Sargassium in 1kg of yellow (*i.e.*, rice) wine for 7 days.

Method of administration: Take 15ml each time, 3 times per day.

General Index

A

B

65, 68, 71
liver/stomach qi pain 225, 226
lockjaw 141, 178
low back aching and pain 34
low back and knee damp heat pain, serious 129
low back and knee aching and pain, kidney vacuity 88
low back and knee chilly pain 49, 86, 93, 137
low back and knee contracture and spasm 144
low back and knee soreness and weakness 37, 50, 52, 55, 67, 69, 37, 50, 52, 55, 67, 69, 85
low back and knees, *bi* pain of the 101
low back and knees, lack of strength of 95
low back and knees, soreness and fatigue of the 203
low back and knees, spasms and cramps in the sinews and vessels of the 92
low back and knees, vacuity chill of 133
low back and leg atony and weakness 124
low back and legs, heaviness of the 166
low back and lower leg aching and pain, wind damp 119
low back and lower leg *bi* and weakness, prolonged summer 83
low back and lower leg *bi* pain 80
low back and lower legs, chilly *bi* of the 97
low back and lower legs, soreness and pain of the 98
low back pain 35, 43, 64, 72, 35, 43, 64, 72, 96, 100, 102, 104, 106, 126, 146, 150, 211
low back pain due to injury from lifting a heavy object 96
low back pain due to prolonged lying on damp earth 72, 96
low back pain, kidney vacuity 35, 43, 35, 43, 96, 102, 106
low back pain, wind cold 96
low back pain, wind toxin 211
low back region, aching and pain in the 99

low back soreness 31, 40, 46, 53, 60, 68, 31, 40, 46, 53, 60, 68
lower abdominal aching and pain 181
lower back and lower extremity aching and pain 175
lower back and lower limb weakness 65
lower leg and foot heaviness, aching, and pain 120
lower leg and foot swelling and fullness 155
lower leg, swelling and distention of the foot and 124
lower legs, wind toxin weak 157
lower origin, chilly vacuity of the 57, 65, 71, 85
lung abscess 5, 156
lung heat coughing and wheezing 216
lung qi upward counterflow 216
lung yin vacuity cough and asthma 36
lung *yong* 205
lung/kidney dual vacuity 64
lung/kidney yin deficiency 44
lupus 4, 79

M

malarial disease 158
male sterility 43
Mao Ze-dong 19
mastitis 169, 213
measles rash 204, 208
measles rash, wind toxin 204
meat, accumulation and stagnation of 167
memory, poor 38, 53, 58, 60, 63, 66, 72, 73, 38, 53, 58, 60, 63, 66, 72, 73, 121, 228
menstrual irregularity 37, 70, 37, 70, 170, 178, 225
menstruation, excessive 179
miasmic qi, invasion of, in tropical regions 191
miasmic toxins, invasions of tropical and mountain 192
miscarriage, incomplete 170
miscarriage, threatened 174

237

Formula Index

A

Acanthopanax & Salvia Wine 100
Achyranthes & Acanthopanax Wine 100
Achyranthes & Aconite Wine 87
Achyranthes & Atractylodes Wine 91
Achyranthes & Cinnamon Wine 85
Achyranthes & Dendrobium Wine 81
Achyranthes & Ginseng Wine 84
Achyranthes & Salvia Wine 83
Achyranthes Compound Wine 102
Aconite & Atractylodes Wine 126
Aconite & Cinnabar Wine 124
Aconite & Eucommia Wine 96
Aconite Wine 87, 104, 116, 122, 123, 131, 139, 163, 164
Acorus & Cinnamon Wine 223
Acorus Wine 17, 121, 172
Acronychia Stem Wine 190
Agkistrodon Wine 210
Allium & Fermented Soybean Wine 186
American Ginseng Wine 51
Amomum Wine 165
Angelica Anomala Wine 180
Angelica Pubescens & Achyranthes Wine 119
Angelica Pubescens & Aconite Wine 123
Angelica Pubescens & Dang Gui Wine 119
Angelica Pubescens & Dendrobium Wine 118
Angelica Pubescens & Ginseng Wine 177
Angelica Pubescens & Loranthus Wine 132
Angelica Pubescens & Notopterygium Wine 115
Angelica Pubescens, Codonopsis & Aconite Wine 116
Arctium & Rehmannia Wine 203
Asarum & Angelica Pubescens Wine 117
Astragalus & Dang Gui Wine 72
Astragalus & Dendrobium Wine 80
Astragalus & Dipsacus Wine 127
Astragalus & Eucommia Wine 89
Astragalus & Ledebouriella Wine 175

Astragalus Wine 33, 90, 111, 112, 179
Atractylodes & Fermented Soybean Wine 156
Atractylodes Wine 45, 91, 126, 128, 164, 174
Atractylodes, Poria & Caulis Lonicerae Wine 166

B

Black Soybean & Angelica Wine 134
Black Soybean & Cinnamon Wine 182
Black Soybean & Salvia Wine 134
Black Soybean Supplement the Kidneys Wine 106
Black Soybean Wine 114, 177
Black Stripe Snake Wine 136
Boost the Kidneys, Brighten the Eyes Wine 68
Boost the Spleen Wine 162
Boosting Longevity Wine 53
Boosting Seed Medicinal Wine 32
Buddha's Hand Wine 196, 224
Burdock Root & Pine Node Wine 155

C

Cannabis Wine 221
Cao Wu Aconite Wine 131
Carthamus Wine 169, 183, 206
Chrysanthemum & Lycium Regulate the Origin Wine 65
Chrysanthemum Wine 82, 153, 185, 227
Chuan Wu Aconite & Eucommia Wine 96
Cibotium Wine 94
Cinnamon & Astragalus Wine 112
Cirsius & Cephalanoplos Wine 173
Cistanches Strengthening Wine 71
Citrus & Gentiana Macrophylla Wine 201
Citrus & Salvia Wine 208
Coix & Achyranthes Wine 143
Coix & Ampelopsis Wine 142
Coix & Dendrobium Wine 103

239

T

V, W, X

OTHER BOOKS ON CHINESE MEDICINE
AVAILABLE FROM BLUE POPPY PRESS
1775 Linden Ave, Boulder, CO 80304
For ordering 1-800-487-9296 PH. 303\447-8372 FAX 303\447-0740

A NEW AMERICAN ACUPUNC-TURE by Mark Seem, ISBN 0-936185-44-9

ACUPUNCTURE AND MOXI-BUSTION FORMULAS & TREAT-MENTS by Cheng Dan-an, trans. by Wu Ming, ISBN 0-936185-68-6

ACUTE ABDOMINAL SYN-DROMES: Their Diagnosis & Treatment by Combined Chinese-Western Medicine by Alon Marcus, ISBN 0-936185-31-7

AGING & BLOOD STASIS: A New Approach to TCM Geriatrics by Yan De-xin, ISBN 0-936185-63-5

AIDS & ITS TREATMENT ACCORDING TO TRADITIONAL CHINESE MEDICINE by Huang Bing-shan, trans. by Fu-Di & Bob Flaws, ISBN 0-936185-28-7

THE BOOK OF JOOK: Chinese Medicinal Porridges, An Alterna-tive to the Typical Western Break-fast by B. Flaws, ISBN0-936185-60-0

CHINESE MEDICAL PALMIS-TRY: Your Health in Your Hand by Zong Xiao-fan & Gary Liscum, ISBN 0-936185-64-3

CHINESE MEDICINAL TEAS: Simple, Proven, Folk Formulas for Common Diseases & Promoting Health by Zong Xiao-fan & Gary Liscum, ISBN 0-936185-76-7

CHINESE MEDICINAL WINES & ELIXIRS by Bob Flaws, ISBN 0-936185-58-9

CHINESE PEDIATRIC MAS-SAGE THERAPY: *A Parent's & Practitioner's Guide to the Prevention & Treatment of Childhood Illness* by Fan Ya-li, ISBN 0-936185-54-6

CHINESE SELF-MASSAGE THE-RAPY: The Easy Way to Health by Fan Ya-li ISBN 0-936185-74-0

CLASSICAL MOXIBUSTION SKILLS in Clinical Practice by Sung Baek, ISBN 0-936185-16-3

A COMPENDIUM OF TCM PAT-TERNS & TREATMENTS by Bob Flaws & Daniel Finney, ISBN 0-936185-70-8

CURING ARTHRITIS NATURALLY WITH CHINESE MEDICINE by Douglas Frank & Bob Flaws ISBN 0-936185-87-2

CURING HAY FEVER NATURALLY WITH CHINESE MEDICINE by Bob Flaws, ISBN 0-936185-91-0

CURING INSOMNIA NATURALLY WITH CHINESE MEDICINE by Bob Flaws ISBN 0-936185-85-6

CURING PMS NATURALLY WITH CHINESE MEDICINE by Bob Flaws ISBN 0-936185-85-6

THE DAO OF INCREASING LONGEVITY AND CONSER-VING ONE'S LIFE by Anna Lin & Bob Flaws, ISBN 0-936185-24-4

THE DAO OF HEALTHY EATING
ACCORDING TO CHINESE
MEDICINE by Bob Flaws, ISBN 0-
936185-92-9

THE DIVINELY RESPONDING
CLASSIC: *A Translation of the Shen Ying
Jing from Zhen Jiu Da Cheng*, trans. by Yang
Shou-zhong & Liu Feng-ting ISBN 0-936185-55-4

DUI YAO: THE ART OF
COMBINING CHINESE HERBAL
MEDICINALS by Philippe Sionneau
ISBN 0-936185-81-3

ENDOMETRIOSIS, INFER-
TILITY AND TRADITIONAL
CHINESE MEDICINE: A
Laywoman's Guide by Bob Flaws ISBN
0-936185-14-7

EXTRA TREATISES BASED ON
INVESTIGATION & INQUIRY: *A
Translation of Zhu Dan-xi's Ge Zhi Yu
Lun*, by Yang Shou-zhong & Duan Wu-jin,
ISBN 0-936185-53-8

FIRE IN THE VALLEY: TCM
Diagnosis & Treatment of Vaginal
Diseases ISBN 0-936185-25-2

FLESHING OUT THE BONES: The
Importance of Case Histories in Chin.
Med. trans. by Chip Chace. ISBN 0-936185-30-9

FU QING-ZHU'S GYNECOLOGY
trans. by Yang Shou-zhong and Liu Da-wei,
ISBN 0-936185-35-X

FULFILLING THE ESSENCE: A
*Handbook of Traditional & Contemporary
Treatments for Female Infertility* by Bob
Flaws, ISBN 0-936185-48-1

GOLDEN NEEDLE WANG LE-
TING: A 20th Century Master's
Approach to Acupuncture by Yu Hui-
chan and Han Fu-ru, trans. by Shuai Xue-zhong,

A HANDBOOK OF TRADI-
TIONAL CHINESE DERMATOL-
OGY by Liang Jian-hui, trans. by Zhang &
Flaws, ISBN 0-936185-07-4

A HANDBOOK OF TRADITION-
AL CHINESE GYNECOLOGY by
Zhejiang College of TCM, trans. by Zhang Ting-
liang, ISBN 0-936185-06-6 (4th edit.)

A HANDBOOK OF MENSTRUAL
DISEASES IN CHINESE MEDI-
CINE by Bob Flaws ISBN 0-936185-82-1

A HANDBOOK of TCM PEDIA-
TRICS by Bob Flaws, ISBN 0-936185-72-4

A HANDBOOK OF TCM UROL-
OGY & MALE SEXUAL DYS-
FUNCTION by Anna Lin, OMD, ISBN 0-
936185-36-8

THE HEART & ESSENCE OF
DAN-XI'S METHODS OF TREAT-
MENT by Xu Dan-xi, trans. by Yang, ISBN 0-
926185-49-X

THE HEART TRANSMISSION OF
MEDICINE by Liu Yi-ren, trans. by Yang
Shou-zhong ISBN 0-936185-83-X

HIGHLIGHTS OF ANCIENT
ACUPUNCTURE PRESCRIP-
TIONS trans. by Wolfe & Crescenz ISBN 0-
936185-23-6

How to Have A HEALTHY PREG-
NANCY, HEALTHY BIRTH with
Chinese Medicine by Honora Lee Wolfe,
ISBN 0-936185-40-6

HOW TO WRITE A TCM HER-
BAL FORMULA: *A Logical Methodology for the Formulation & Administration
of Chinese Herbal Medicine in Decoction*
by Bob Flaws, ISBN 0-936185-49-X

IMPERIAL SECRETS OF
HEALTH & LONGEVITY by Bob
Flaws, ISBN 0-936185-51-1

KEEPING YOUR CHILD HEAL-
THY WITH CHINESE MEDICINE
by Bob Flaws, ISBN 0-936185-71-6

Li Dong-yuan's TREATISE ON
THE SPLEEN & STOMACH, *A*
Translation of the Pi Wei Lun by Yang
Shou-zhong & Li Jian-yong, ISBN 0-936185-41-4

LOW BACK PAIN: Care & Prevention with Chinese Medicine by Douglas
Frank, ISBN 0-936185-66-X

MASTER HUA'S CLASSIC OF
THE CENTRAL VISCERA by Hua
Tuo, ISBN 0-936185-43-0

MASTER TONG'S ACUPUNC-
TURE: An Ancient Alternative
Style in Modern Clinical Practice by
Miriam Lee, ISBN 0-936185-37-6

THE MEDICAL I CHING: *Oracle*
of the Healer Within by Miki Shima, OMD,
ISBN 0-936185-38-4

MENOPAUSE A Second Spring:
Making a Smooth Transition with
Chinese Medicine by Honora Lee Wolfe
ISBN 0-936185-18-X

PAO ZHI: Introduction to Process-
ing Chinese Medicinals to Enhance
Their Therapeutic Effect, by Philippe
Sionneau, ISBN 0-936185-62-1

PATH OF PREGNANCY, VOL. I,
Gestational Disorders by Bob Flaws,
ISBN 0-936185-39-2
PATH OF PREGNANCY, Vol. II,
Postpartum Diseases by Bob Flaws. ISBN
0-936185-42-2

PEDIATRIC BRONCHITIS: Its
Cause, Diagnosis & Treatment Ac-
cording to TCM trans. by Gao Yu-li and
Bob Flaws, ISBN 0-936185-26-0

PRINCE WEN HUI'S COOK: Chi-
nese Dietary Therapy by Bob Flaws &
Honora Lee Wolfe, ISBN 0-912111-05-4, $12.95
(Published by Paradigm Press)

THE PULSE CLASSIC: A Translation of the *Mai Jing* by Wang Shu-he,
trans. by Yang Shou-zhong ISBN 0-936185-75-9

RECENT TCM RESEARCH
FROM CHINA, trans. by Charles Chace &
Bob Flaws, ISBN 0-936185-56-2
SCATOLOGY & THE GATE OF
LIFE: The Large Intestine in Immu-
nity by Bob Flaws ISBN 0-936185-20-1

THE SECRET OF CHINESE
PULSE DIAGNOSIS by Bob Flaws,
ISBN 0-936185-67-8

SEVENTY ESSENTIAL TCM
FORMULAS FOR BEGINNERS by
Bob Flaws, ISBN 0-936185-59-7

SHAOLIN SECRET FORMULAS
for Treatment of External Injuries,
by De Chan, ISBN 0-936185-08-2

STATEMENTS OF FACT IN
TRADITIONAL CHINESE MEDI-
CINE by Bob Flaws, ISBN 0-936185-52-X,

STICKING TO THE POINT: A
Rational Methodology for the Step
by Step Formulation & Administration of an Acupuncture Treatment
by Bob Flaws ISBN 0-936185-17-1

THE SYSTEMATIC CLASSIC OF
ACUPUNCTURE & MOXIBUS-
TION (*Jia Yi Jing*) by Huang-fu Mi, trans. by
Yang Shou-zhong & Charles Chace, ISBN 0-
936185-29-5

THE TREATMENT OF DISEASE
IN TCM, Vol I: Diseases of the Head
& Face Including Mental/Emotional
Disorders by Philippe Sionneau & Lü Gang,
ISBN 0-936185-69-4

THE TREATMENT OF DISEASE IN TCM, Vol. II: Diseases of the Eyes, Ears, Nose, & Throat by Sionneau & Lü, ISBN 0-936185-69-4

THE TREATMENT OF DISEASE, VOL. III: Diseases of the Mouth, Lips, Tongue, Teeth & Gums, by Sionneau & Lü, ISBN 0-936185-79-1

THE TREATMENT OF DISEASE, VOL VI: Diseases of the Neck, Shoulders, Upper & Lower Back, & Extremities, by Philippe Sionneau & Lü Gang, ISBN 0-936185-89-9

THE TREATMENT OF EXTERNAL DISEASES WITH ACUPUNCTURE & MOXIBUSTION by Yan Cui-lan and Zhu Yun-long, ISBN 0-936185-80-5